NSNA Review

Gerontologic Nursing

Consulting Editor
Ann M. Carignan, R.N.C., M.S.N.
Professor of Nursing
Valencia Community College
Department of Nursing
Orlando, Florida

Reviewers
Amy B. Sharron, R.N., M.S., C.R.N.P.
Geriatric Nurse Practitioner and Instructor of Nursing
The Pennsylvania State University
School of Nursing
University Park, Pennsylvania

Wanda May Webb, R.N., M.S.N.
Level Coordinator and Instructor
Brandywine School of Nursing
Coatesville, Pennsylvania
Staff Nurse
Hickory House Nursing Home
Honey Brook, Pennsylvania

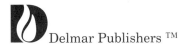
Delmar Publishers ™

I(T)P· An International Thomson Publishing Company

Albany • Bonn • Boston • Cinncinati • Detroit • London • Madrid • Melbourne
Mexico City • New York • Pacific Grove • Paris • San Francisco • Singapore • Tokyo
Toronto • Washington

Developed for Delmar Publishers Inc. by Visual Education Corporation, Princeton, New Jersey.
Publisher: David Gordon
Sponsoring Editor: Patricia Casey
Project Director: Susan J. Garver
Developmental Editor: Cynthia E. Mooney
Production Supervisor: Amy Davis
Production Assistant: Kristen Walczak
Proofreading Management: William A. Murray
Word Processing: Cynthia C. Feldner
Composition: Maxson Crandall, Lisa Evans-Skopas, Christine Osborne
Cover Designer: Paul C. Uhl, DESIGNASSOCIATES
Text Designer: Circa 86

Copyright © 1995

By Delmar Publishers
a division of International Thomson Publishing Inc.

The ITP logo is a trademark under license.

Printed in the United States of America

For more information contact:

Delmar Publishers
3 Columbia Circle, Box 15015
Albany, New York 12212-5015

Delmar Publishers' Online Services
To access Delmar on the World Wide Web, point your browser to:
http://www.delmar.com/delmar.html
To access through Gopher: gopher://gopher.delmar.com
(Delmar Online is part of "thomson.com", an internet site with information on
more than 30 publishers of the International Thomson Publishing organization.)
For information on our products and services:
email: info@delmar.com
or call 800-347-7707

International Thomson Publishing
Europe
Berkshire House 168-173
High Holborn
London, WCIV 7AA
England

Thomas Nelson Australia
102 Dodds Street
South Melbourne, 3205
Victoria, Australia

Nelson Canada
1120 Birchmont Road
Scarborough, Ontario
Canada, M1K 5G4

International Thomson Editores
Campos Eliscos 385, Piso 7
Col Polanco
11560 Mexico D F Mexico

International Thomson Publishing GmbH
Konigswinterer Strasse 418
53227 Bonn, Germany

International Thomson Publishing Asia
#05-10 Henderson Building
221 Henderson Road
Singapore 0315

International Thomson Publishing Japan
Hirakawacho Kyowa Building, 3F
2-2-1 Hirakawacho
Chiyoda-ku, Tokyo 102
Japan

2 3 4 5 6 7 8 9 10 XXX 00 99 98 97 96

Library of Congress Cataloging-in-Publication Data

Gerontologic nursing / consulting editor, Ann M. Carignan; reviewers Amy B. Sharron,
    Wanda May Webb.
        p. cm. — (NASA review series)
    Developed for Delmar Publishers Inc. by Visual Education Corporation.
    ISBN 0-8273-6484-9
    1. Geriatric nursing—Outlines, syllabi, etc.   I. Carignan, Ann M.   II. National Student Nurses'
Association (U.S.)   III. Visual Education Corporation.   IV. Series.
    [DNLM: 1. Geriatric Nursing—outlines. WY 18 G3762 1995]
    RC954.G4734 1995
    610.73´65—dc20
    DNLM/DLC   94-31990
    for Library of Congress   CIP

Titles in Series

Maternal-Newborn Nursing

Pediatric Nursing

Nursing Pharmacology

Medical-Surgical Nursing

Psychiatric Nursing

Gerontologic Nursing

Health Assessment and Physical Examination

Community Health Nursing
(available in 1996)

Nutrition and Diet Therapy
(available in 1996)

Series Advisory Board

Series Review Board

Contents

Notice to the Reader

Preface

The NSNA Review Series is a multiple-volume series designed to help nursing students review course content and prepare for course tests.

Chapter elements include:

Overview—lists the main topic headings for the chapter

Nursing Highlights—gives significant nursing care concepts relevant to the chapter

Glossary—features key terms used in the chapter that are not defined within the chapter

Enhanced Outline—consists of short, concise phrases, clauses, and sentences that summarize the main topics of course content; focuses on nursing care and the nursing process; includes the following elements:
- *Client Teaching Checklists:* shaded boxes that feature important issues to discuss with clients; designed to help students prepare client education sections of nursing care plans
- *Nurse Alerts:* shaded boxes that provide information that is of critical importance to the nurse, such as danger signs or emergency measures connected with a particular condition or situation
- *Locators:* finding aids placed across the top of the page that indicate the main outline section that is being covered on a particular 2-page spread within the context of other main section heads
- *Textbook reference aids:* boxes labeled "See text pages ____," which appear in the margin next to each main head, to be used by students to list the page numbers in their textbook that cover the material presented in that section of the outline
- *Cross references:* references to other parts of the outline, which identify the relevant section of the outline by using the numbered and lettered outline levels (e.g., "same as section I,A,1,b" or "see section II,B,3")

Chapter Tests—review and reinforce chapter material through questions in a format similar to that of the National Council Licensure Examination for Registered Nurses (NCLEX-RN); answers follow the questions and contain rationales for both correct and incorrect answers

Comprehensive Test—appears at the end of the book and includes items that review material from each chapter

1

Health Promotion and the Elderly Client

OVERVIEW

I. Theories of aging
- A. Physiologic and biologic theories
- B. Psychosocial theories

II. Theories of human development associated with aging
- A. Erik Erikson
- B. Robert Peck

III. Basic concepts of gerontologic nursing
- A. History
- B. Theoretic framework
- C. Primary nursing responsibilities

IV. Promoting cardiac function
- A. Risk factors for impaired cardiac function
- B. Nursing interventions

V. Promoting ventilation
- A. Risk factors for impaired ventilation
- B. Nursing interventions

VI. Promoting adequate nutrition
- A. Risk factors for impaired nutrition
- B. Nursing interventions

VII. Promoting integumentary function
- A. Risk factors for abnormal integumentary function
- B. Nursing interventions

VIII. Promoting normal excretory patterns
- A. Risk factors for abnormal excretory patterns
- B. Nursing interventions

IX. Promoting sufficient activity levels
- A. Risk factors for inadequate activity
- B. Nursing interventions

X. Promoting sufficient amounts of sleep
- A. Risk factors for impaired sleep
- B. Nursing interventions

XI. Promoting appropriate social interaction
- A. Risk factors that impair social interaction
- B. Nursing interventions

XII. Promoting appropriate sexuality
- A. Risk factors to sexuality
- B. Nursing interventions

XIII. Promoting safety
- A. Risk factors to safety
- B. Nursing interventions

NURSING HIGHLIGHTS

1. The process of aging is influenced by many factors, such as heredity and environment, that contribute to different manifestations of aging patterns in different individuals.
2. It is the role of the gerontologic nurse to promote and maintain the health and self-care practices of the aging client as well as to care for those elderly clients who have health problems.

GLOSSARY

debridement—removal of damaged necrotic tissue from a pressure sore or skin ulcer

free radical—a highly reactive molecule produced during oxygen metabolism that can damage proteins, enzymes, and DNA

functional incontinence—inability or unwillingness to void because the individual is unaware of the need to urinate or cannot reach a toilet; often associated with severe cognitive disorders, physical disabilities, or environmental barriers

homeostasis—a relative constancy in the body's internal environment, maintained through adaptive responses

lipofuscin—a member of a group of insoluble fatty pigments formed by the solution of pigment in fat

nocturia—the need, usually excessive, to urinate at night

overflow incontinence—leakage of urine because pressure resulting from a chronically full bladder exceeds urethral resistance; often associated with benign prostatic hypertrophy, strictures, fecal impaction, and some medications

stress incontinence—involuntary loss of urine because intra-abdominal pressure is greater than urethral resistance; often associated with coughing, sneezing, laughing, or heavy lifting

urge incontinence—involuntary loss of the ability to hold urine long enough to reach the toilet after the immediate urge to urinate is felt; often associated with disorders of the central nervous system

ENHANCED OUTLINE

See text pages
_____

I. Theories of aging

A. Physiologic and biologic theories
  1. Genetic theories: Aging is under genetic control and occurs at the cell level.
    a) Cellular mutations occur as a result of exposure to radiation or chemicals and cause organ damage.

b) The ability of RNA to synthesize and translate messages becomes impaired in the elderly person.

c) An aging factor that contributes to cell maturation becomes active or is produced in excessive quantities in the older adult.

d) Cell growth and reproduction cease when a critical growth factor is used up or stops being produced.

2. Cross-link theory: Cell division becomes impaired, and cell death occurs.

a) Chemical bonds are created between structures that are normally separate.

b) Normal parting of DNA strands during mitosis is prevented.

3. Free-radical theory: Cumulative damage from free-radical molecules gradually causes physical deterioration.

4. Accumulation of lipofuscin: Accumulation interferes with transport of metabolites and information-bearing molecules within cells.

5. Immunologic theory: A lessening of immunologic activities occurs during aging that leads to enhanced autoimmune response and tissue damage.

6. Stress and adaptation theories: Aging-related changes reduce the body's ability to restore homeostasis in the presence of stress. Stress depletes adaptive ability; in turn, body's reduced adaptive capacity may lead to more stress.

B. Psychosocial theories

1. Disengagement theory: Society and the older person gradually withdraw from each other. The withdrawal is satisfactory to both.

2. Activity theory: Physical, social, and economic activities should be maintained during the later years. Self-concept is related to the roles one holds.

3. Continuity theory: Ideas, habits, and coping abilities developed over a lifetime determine whether a person remains engaged and active or becomes disengaged and inactive during old age.

II. Theories of human development associated with aging

See text pages
_____

A. Erik Erikson

1. Humans must achieve balance between the following tasks during each stage of development in order to grow throughout the life span.

a) Trust versus mistrust: infancy

b) Autonomy versus shame and doubt: early childhood

c) Initiative versus guilt: late childhood

d) Industry versus inferiority: school age

e) Identity versus role diffusion: adolescence

f) Intimacy versus isolation: young adulthood

g) Generativity versus stagnation: adulthood

h) Integrity versus despair: old age (age 65–death)

2. Basic attitudes associated with integrity are wisdom and acceptance of the value of one's life.

3. Basic attitudes associated with despair are sense of loss, criticism of and contempt for others, and worry over past mistakes.

B. Robert Peck: challenges for the elderly
1. Ego differentiation versus role preoccupation: finding personal satisfaction apart from job and children
2. Body transcendence versus body preoccupation: avoiding preoccupation with minor physical ailments
3. Ego transcendence versus ego preoccupation: overcoming preoccupation with death by helping younger generation

III. Basic concepts of gerontologic nursing

See text pages
_____

A. History
1. Gerontologic nursing evolved as a discipline during the early part of the 20th century as the number of residential care facilities for the elderly began to increase.
2. In 1966 the Geriatric Nursing Division of the American Nurses Association (ANA) was formed (renamed Gerontological Nursing Division in 1976).
3. Standards of Gerontological Nursing Practice (originally called Standards of Geriatric Nursing) was first published in 1970 by the ANA and is periodically revised.
4. The first nurses were certified in gerontologic nursing in 1975 by the ANA.

B. Theoretic framework: All nursing practice should be based on an appropriate theoretic framework.
1. Orem's self-care theory (see also section IV,C of Chapter 2)
   a) All individuals have universal life demands (e.g., air, water, food, excretion, activity, rest, social interaction, solitude, avoidance of hazards, maintenance of normalcy).
   b) Each person has unique capabilities and shortcomings in meeting those demands.
   c) Self-care capacity is the ability to take responsibility for meeting those needs.
   d) A self-care limitation occurs when a person is partially or totally unable to fulfill a need.
   e) The basis of nursing actions involves helping the client maintain functional independence by encouraging capabilities and reducing limitations.
2. Roy's adaptation theory
   a) Over the course of life, a person executes positive and negative adaptations to internal and external environments.
   b) Adaptations occur in the areas of basic physiologic needs, self-concept, role function, and interdependence relations during health and illness.

      c) The basis of nursing actions involves predicting stressful events and helping the client cope with them.
   3. Wellness theory
      a) Wellness is a balance between an individual's internal and external environment and his/her emotional, spiritual, social, cultural, and physical processes.
      b) Gerontologic nursing involves the concepts of health promotion, health maintenance, disease prevention, and self-care as well as a focus on illness.
      c) Nursing actions include assessment, intervention, education, referral, and evaluation.

C. Primary nursing responsibilities
   1. Strengthening the client's self-care capacities
   2. Eliminating or minimizing the client's self-care limitations
   3. Providing direct services by assisting the client when demands cannot be adequately fulfilled

IV. Promoting cardiac function

See text pages _____

A. Risk factors for impaired cardiac function
   1. Positive family history
   2. High intake of animal fat, salt, and calories
   3. Obesity
   4. Cigarette smoking
   5. Lack of exercise
   6. Sustained exposure to stress and internalizing of emotions
   7. Exposure to environmental and occupational toxins
   8. The presence of chronic conditions, such as anemia, cardiac arrhythmias, diabetes, hypertension, infection, malnutrition, and renal disease

B. Nursing interventions
   1. Encourage the client to adhere to current dietary guidelines regarding intake of fats, sodium, and calories.
   2. Assist the overweight client in identifying and participating in an appropriate program for gradual weight loss (2–4 lb/month).
   3. Advise the client who smokes cigarettes to stop, perhaps by participating in a smoking cessation class or support group.
   4. Encourage the client to participate in an appropriate exercise program.
      a) Daily passive or active range-of-motion exercises for clients who are confined to bed
      b) Daily organized sessions of arm and leg raising, flexion and extension, kicking, and ball catching for those who use a wheelchair
      c) A daily walk of 1–2 miles (weather permitting)
      d) Swimming, tennis, or golf in moderation, if health level is appropriate

5. Teach the client to try to avoid stressful situations, to use stress-reduction techniques such as progressive relaxation (muscle tensing and relaxing) or guided imagery, and to share concerns with a supportive family member or friend.
6. Caution the client to try to minimize exposure to toxic substances and to be aware of any possible exposures.
7. Advise the client to participate in the management of chronic conditions by keeping appointments, following instructions, and taking medications as they were prescribed.
8. Assist the client in conserving energy and preventing oxygen demand from exceeding functional capacity by efficient organization of the home and work environment, pacing activities, and setting aside time for rest.

V. Promoting ventilation

See text pages
_____

A. Risk factors for impaired ventilation
   1. Reduced efficiency in air expulsion due to age-related physiologic changes
   2. Lowered resistance to infection because of weakened immune system and diminished self-cleaning by respiratory cilia
   3. Presence of small, diffuse areas of lung destruction in generally healthy nonsmokers
   4. Decreased chest expansion due to rib cage rigidity, the presence of kyphosis and scoliosis, and stooped posture
   5. Decreased blood oxygen (PO_2) level
   6. Damage caused by long-term cigarette smoking
   7. Damage caused by exposure to occupational or hobby-related air pollutants

B. Nursing interventions
   1. Prevent respiratory complications by educating the client about prophylactic measures that will lessen the client's susceptibility to respiratory infections, such as receiving annual influenza immunizations and staying away from ill people who may be contagious.
   2. Encourage the client to maintain resistance to illness by eating a balanced diet.
   3. Advise the client to increase fluid intake during respiratory infections to mobilize respiratory secretions.
   4. Encourage the client to pace daily activities to maintain adequate oxygenation and conserve energy.
   5. Teach the client to maintain maximum breathing ability by doing daily breathing exercises (see Client Teaching Checklist, "Deep-Breathing Exercises").
   6. Urge the client to maintain the most erect posture possible.

Deep-Breathing Exercises

Explanations to the client:

Abdominal/diaphragmatic exercises
- ✔ Stand, or lie down with knees bent.
- ✔ Place 1 hand on the abdomen (below ribs) and the other hand on the middle of the chest.
- ✔ Inhale slowly and deeply through the nose, relaxing abdominal muscles and letting the abdomen expand.
- ✔ The hand over the chest should not move; the hand on the abdomen should fall with inhalation and rise with exhalation.
- ✔ Breathe out through pursed lips, contracting the abdominal muscles. Use hand on abdomen to press inward and upward on the abdomen while exhaling. Exhalation should last longer than inhalation. It is important to try to empty the lungs as completely as possible.
- ✔ Do several times a day; start with 1 minute and build up to 5 minutes.

Pursed-lip breathing
- ✔ Breathe in through the nose.
- ✔ Exhale very slowly and evenly through pursed lips, prolonging exhalation. Take longer to exhale than to inhale.
- ✔ Exhale as much air as you can.
- ✔ Use this type of breathing during any exercise activity.

7. Advise the client to humidify his/her living quarters to help keep mucous membranes intact.
8. Encourage the client to avoid stressful situations and use stress-reduction techniques, because emotional stress, anxiety, and fear accelerate respiration and thus increase oxygen demand.
9. When possible, place clients who are confined to bed in the sitting position to optimize chest expansion.
10. Turn recumbent clients frequently from side to side and to the back.
11. Caution clients to limit their exposure to air pollutants, such as the chlorinated hydrocarbons used in many model-building and craft activities.

VI. Promoting adequate nutrition

See text pages
_____

A. Risk factors for impaired nutrition
 1. Age-related decreases in sensations of taste and smell
 2. Inadequate hydration
 3. Poor oral health (e.g., decayed, broken, missing teeth); periodontal disease; ill-fitting dentures; and oral lesions
 4. Poor lifelong food use patterns and ignorance of good nutritional practices

5. Inadequate income
6. Lack of transportation and adequate food storage or preparation facilities
7. Lack of opportunities for socializing while eating
8. Alcoholism and drug abuse
9. Depression, psychosis, and cognitive impairment

B. Nursing interventions
   1. Explain to the client that adequate hydration (2 liters of fluid daily, half of which should be water) is essential to preserve body functions, prevent dehydration, achieve good digestion, maintain skin and mucous membrane integrity, and produce antibodies.
   2. Make sure that the client has a basic understanding of the principles of nutrition, including the suggested daily food choices and appropriate numbers of servings as recommended in Food Guide

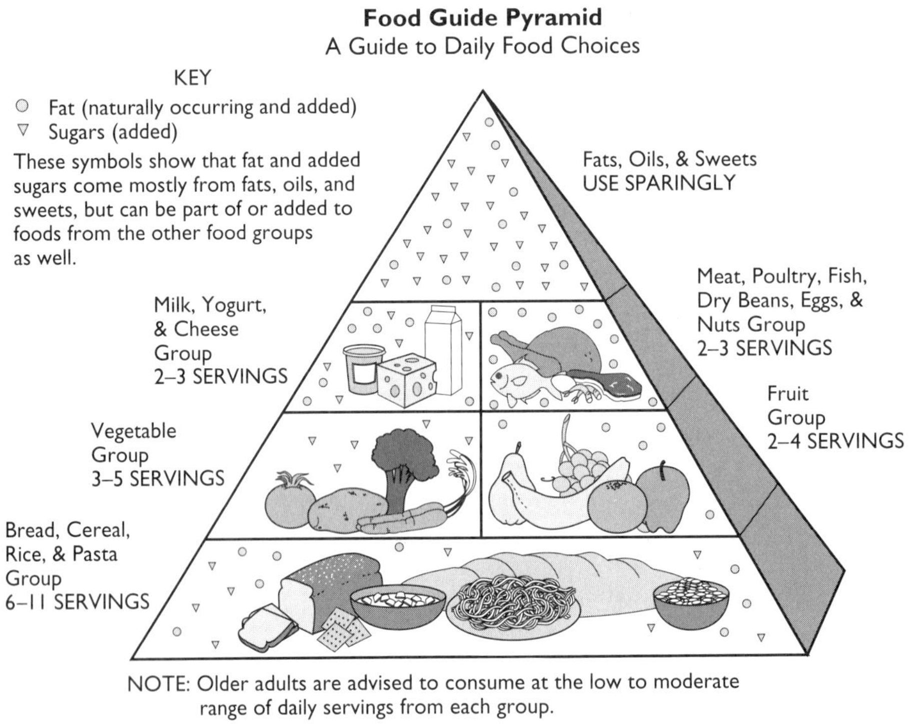

Food Guide Pyramid
A Guide to Daily Food Choices

KEY
○ Fat (naturally occurring and added)
▽ Sugars (added)
These symbols show that fat and added sugars come mostly from fats, oils, and sweets, but can be part of or added to foods from the other food groups as well.

Fats, Oils, & Sweets
USE SPARINGLY

Milk, Yogurt, & Cheese Group
2–3 SERVINGS

Meat, Poultry, Fish, Dry Beans, Eggs, & Nuts Group
2–3 SERVINGS

Vegetable Group
3–5 SERVINGS

Fruit Group
2–4 SERVINGS

Bread, Cereal, Rice, & Pasta Group
6–11 SERVINGS

NOTE: Older adults are advised to consume at the low to moderate range of daily servings from each group.

Figure 1–1
Food Guide Pyramid: A Guide to Daily Food Choices
SOURCE: U.S. Department of Agriculture/U.S. Department of Health and Human Services

Pyramid; the functions of proteins, fats, and carbohydrates; the importance of vitamins and minerals; and the meaning of a calorie.

3. Explain current guidelines for overall dietary intake and recommended intake levels of proteins, carbohydrates, and fats.
4. Caution clients about the unsupervised use of vitamin and mineral supplements, because some vitamins are toxic when taken at excessive doses and many supplements can interact with prescription drugs, causing a variety of adverse reactions.
5. Discuss the basic principles of oral hygiene and help clients obtain access to low-cost dental care.
6. When appropriate, arrange for a clinical nutritional assessment to look for signs and symptoms of nutritional deficiencies; take anthropometric measurements, including weight, stature, and skinfolds; and analyze hematologic and biochemical parameters (see Nurse Alert, "Recognizing the Signs of Nutritional Deficiencies").
7. Teach clients the dangers associated with obesity, including an increased risk for cardiovascular disease and diabetes and the exacerbation of musculoskeletal problems, such as arthritis.
8. Explain to clients that excessive cholesterol intake (more than 300 mg/day) is associated with heart disease, stroke, and cancer.
9. If not contraindicated because of an existing condition, advise clients to consume 25–35 g of fiber daily by eating vegetables, whole grain products, and fruits.

! NURSE *ALERT* !

Recognizing the Signs of Nutritional Deficiencies

It has been estimated that at least 30% of noninstitutionalized elderly people have a significant deficit of at least 1 important dietary nutrient. It is important to recognize the manifestations of nutritional deficiencies.

Adverse effects/manifestations of vitamin deficiencies
- Vitamin A: dermatitis, impaired night vision
- Vitamin B_1: malaise, anorexia, weakness in the legs, burning feet, palpitations, heart failure
- Vitamin B_2: burning eyes, misty vision, hair loss
- Vitamin B_3: irritability, forgetfulness, depression, peripheral neuropathy
- Vitamin B_{12}: neurologic changes, inflammation of the tongue
- Vitamin C: gingivitis, bleeding gums, spontaneous bruising, arthralgia
- Folic acid: forgetfulness, irritability, paranoid behavior, anorexia

Adverse effects/manifestations of mineral deficiencies
- Calcium and phosphorus: repeated fractures, generalized pain
- Fluoride: dental caries
- Zinc: hair loss; impaired taste, smell, night vision; delayed wound healing

10. Urge clients to consume calcium (800 mg/day for males, 1000 mg/day for females taking estrogen, 1500 mg/day for females not on estrogen) and to get sufficient exercise to prevent or delay the progress of osteoporosis. Foods such as milk, yogurt, cheese, vegetables, greens, fish, and nuts are good sources of calcium.
11. Caution clients about the dangers of quick weight-loss diets.
12. Advise clients that high alcohol intake contributes to vitamin B_1 and B_3 deficiency, damages organs required for nutrient absorption and use, and causes anorexia.

VII. Promoting integumentary function

See text pages
_____

A. Risk factors for abnormal integumentary function
1. Dry skin (xerosis), reflecting abnormalities of epidermal maturation caused by cumulative skin injuries and aggravated by nutritional deficiencies and exposure to cold temperatures, dry air, harsh soaps, and hot baths
2. Itching (pruritus) that may be a side effect of a drug or caused by renal failure, hepatic disease, and anemia; may also be aggravated by allergies, sudden temperature changes, extreme heat, perspiration, dry skin, rubbing of clothing, emotional stress, and fatigue
3. Pressure sores caused by tissue ischemia and anoxia and associated with poor nutritional status, extreme thinness, impaired sensory feedback mechanisms, vascular insufficiency, immobility, and corticosteroid therapy
4. Sebaceous or actinic keratosis or squamous cell or basal cell carcinoma; usually associated with prolonged exposure to the sun over many years
5. Skin ulcerations of the extremities caused by vascular insufficiency

B. Nursing interventions
1. Encourage the client with dry skin to rehydrate the dermis by using superfatted soaps (Basis, Dove), lotions, and emollients; humidifying the home; avoiding hot baths; limiting the total number of baths or showers to 1–2 a week; and avoiding tight clothing that rubs against the skin.
2. Advise the client to control itching by rehydrating the skin; using lotions such as Lubriderm; applying cold saline compresses; taking Epsom salt or oatmeal baths; or, in severe cases and if not contraindicated with other medicines or with allergies, taking low doses of an antihistamine at bedtime.
3. Caution the client to avoid scratching the skin or drying it vigorously with a towel. Suggest that the client apply lotion when skin is still slightly damp.

4. Prevent or minimize pressure sores by turning the immobile client at least every 2 hours, gently massaging bony areas, lifting rather than dragging or sliding the client, and helping the client maintain a diet high in carbohydrates, proteins, and vitamins.
5. Treat pressure sores with transparent film or hydrocolloid wafer dressings, Gelfoam, chemical debridement, Karaya powder, absorption dressings, or wet-to-dry dressings; surgical debridement may be performed by a physician in severe cases.
6. Urge clients with skin lesions to consult a physician for evaluation, treatment, and removal.
7. Encourage clients with vascular insufficiency to prevent skin ulceration by attending to injuries of the lower extremities and wearing elastic stockings to enhance circulation.
8. Treat vascular ulcers of the extremities with bed rest; elevation of the legs while sitting; application of topical antibiotics, normal saline solution, or Burow's compresses or soaks; or chemical debridement agents; surgical debridement may be performed by a physician in severe cases.

VIII. Promoting normal excretory patterns

See text pages
_____

A. Risk factors for abnormal excretory patterns
   1. Urinary incontinence: functional incontinence, overflow incontinence, stress incontinence, urge incontinence
      a) Decreased bladder volume
      b) Increased urinary frequency and urgency
      c) Severe illness (e.g., cerebrovascular disease)
      d) Difficulty in walking, unfastening clothing, or handling a urinal or bedpan
      e) Emotional disturbances or dementia
      f) Prescription of drugs that increase urinary output (e.g., diuretics) or those that produce drowsiness or confusion (e.g., sedatives, tranquilizers, hypnotics)
      g) Prolapsed bladder
   2. Bowel problems
      a) Constipation caused by consumption of a low-fiber diet, insufficient consumption of fluids, laxative abuse, diminished muscle tone and motor function, impairment of the defecation reflex, poor toileting habits, and postponed passage of stool
      b) Fecal impaction caused by unrecognized or untreated constipation
      c) Fecal incontinence caused by cerebrovascular disease, severe arteriosclerosis, neurologic impairment, muscular flaccidity, administration of certain medications (antibiotics, digitalis, iron supplements), inability to get to the toilet, prolonged laxative dependence, insufficient dietary fiber, inadequate fluid intake, lack of exercise, hemorrhoids, and depression

VI. Promoting adequate nutrition	VII. Promoting integumentary function	VIII. Promoting excretory patterns	IX. Promoting sufficient activity levels	X. Promoting sufficient amounts of sleep

B. Nursing interventions
  1. Urinary incontinence
    a) Perform a complete physical workup, including bladder function tests, to determine appropriate treatment.
    b) Ensure that the client has access to a toilet or to an appropriate toilet substitute (e.g., commode, overtoilet chair, bedpan, urinal) and that the client has privacy.
    c) Teach the client how to use protective undergarments.
    d) Instruct the client with urge or stress incontinence in the use of behavioral techniques intended to enhance awareness of the lower urinary tract (e.g., habit training, scheduled toileting, bladder retraining, biofeedback, pelvic muscle exercises, Kegel exercises).
    e) Protect the skin of incontinent clients by frequent inspection for wetness, washing and thoroughly drying skin that has come into contact with urine, and application of a thin layer of ointment or skin lubricant.
    f) Administer drugs as prescribed for incontinence (e.g., flavoxate, oxybutynin, pseudoephedrine).
    g) Discuss with clients the surgical interventions sometimes used to treat urinary incontinence (e.g., suspension of the bladder neck, prostatectomy, sphincter implantation, bladder augmentation).
    h) Use Foley and condom catheters only as a last resort.
  2. Bowel problems
    a) Explain to clients that constipation is the diminished frequency of elimination that represents a change in bowel habits. Emphasize that failure to have a daily bowel movement does not necessarily indicate the presence of constipation.
    b) Encourage the client with constipation to eat a high-fiber diet, drink at least 2 liters of fluid per day, drink senna tea rather than taking over-the-counter laxatives, get adequate exercise (e.g., passive or active range of motion, pelvic tilt, walking), and place the feet on a stool during evacuation.
    c) Manually remove fecal impactions after softening them with multiple enemas or an oil-retention enema.
    d) Prevent further impaction by ensuring that the client consumes at least 2 liters of fluid per day, eats a high-fiber diet, and gets a schedule that allows sufficient time for defecation.
    e) Assist the client with fecal incontinence to manage the problem in a manner consistent with the cause of the disorder and his/her general health and cognitive status: approaches include consuming 6–10 g of dietary fiber per day, identifying triggers that cause incontinence (finishing a meal, drinking coffee), controlling the time(s) of day at which defecation occurs, and wearing protective undergarments.

IX. Promoting sufficient activity levels

See text pages
_____

A. Risk factors for inadequate activity
1. Misconceptions about the level of exertion or the degree of risk involved in healthy exercise, and the idea that exercise is for young people
2. Fear of pain or incontinence
3. Lack of exercise facilities or transportation
4. Changes in joints caused by arthritis
5. Gait problems due to Parkinson's disease, orthostatic hypotension, or hemiparesis
6. Lack of knowledge in correct method of using walker, cane, or other assistive device

B. Nursing interventions
1. Explain the benefits of exercise (see Client Teaching Checklist, "The Benefits of Exercise").
2. Explain the advantages of aerobic exercises (e.g., swimming, cycling, brisk walking).
3. Help the client who is reluctant to exercise alone to identify an appropriate community program.
4. Advise the client to begin each exercise session with warm-ups and to conclude with at least 10 minutes of cool-down exercises.
5. Caution the client to stop exercising immediately if he/she experiences chest pain or pressure, dizziness, breathlessness, or fainting and to tell the physician.

✔ CLIENT TEACHING CHECKLIST ✔

The Benefits of Exercise

Explain these benefits of exercise to the aging client:

Physiologic and functional benefits
- ✔ Reduces age-related declines in respiratory and cardiovascular function
- ✔ Minimizes bone loss, improves bone mineral content, and reduces risk of fracture
- ✔ Improves cardiorespiratory endurance, muscle strength and endurance, balance, agility, and flexibility
- ✔ Facilitates weight maintenance

Psychologic benefits
- ✔ Promotes positive moods, stress reduction, improved self-image
- ✔ Encourages better sleep
- ✔ Enhances cognitive functioning

NOTE: Explain to the client that a thorough physical assessment should precede participation in any exercise program.

6. Advise the client to modify the exercise program if joint pain persists 2 hours after an exercise session.
7. Help the client to obtain appropriate assistive devices, and instruct in proper use.

See text pages

X. Promoting sufficient amounts of sleep

A. Risk factors for impaired sleep
 1. Age-related physiologic factors (e.g., naps during the day, sleep that is less deep than it was, a decrease in total sleep time, an increase in the number of awakenings during the night)
 2. Pathologic factors (e.g., pain, increased gastric secretions, nocturia, sleep apnea)
 3. Side effects of drugs (e.g., tricyclic antidepressants)
 4. Psychologic factors (e.g., anxiety, bereavement, relocation, depression, dementia)

B. Nursing interventions
 1. Explain to the client that sleep is a restorative process during which cell growth and repair take place.
 2. Advise the client that sleep deprivation may lead to lethargy, decreased alertness, increased irritability, and hypersensitivity to pain and cold.
 3. Encourage the client to follow a nightly routine that enhances the quality of sleep, including:
   a) Going to bed and getting up at the same time each day
   b) Following a predictable routine before bed
   c) Drinking a milk-based drink, if desired, because milk contains tryptophan, which increases serotonin levels in the brain and may therefore induce sleep
   d) Practicing relaxation techniques, such as muscle tension/release exercises, meditation, or prayer
   e) Sleeping in a warm, quiet environment on a firm but comfortable mattress
   f) Using the bedroom only for sleeping
 4. With the knowledge of the prescribing physician, suggest that the client take prescribed medications so that they support, rather than interfere with, the process of sleep.
   a) Take an analgesic just before bed to minimize the chance of awakening due to pain.
   b) Take diuretics well before bedtime to curtail the need for nighttime urination.
   c) Take antiparkinson drugs and antidepressants at bedtime.

5. Urge the client to avoid stimulating activities and stimulants just before bedtime (e.g., drinking caffeinated beverages or alcohol, smoking, exercising).
6. Caution the client that sleep medications should be taken only on a short-term basis. Most benzodiazepines lose their sleep-promoting properties within 3–14 days, and rebound insomnia may occur when they are discontinued.
7. Explain to the client that because of incomplete excretion, sleeping medication may have a hangover effect during the day and may increase risk of falls.

XI. Promoting appropriate social interaction

See text pages
_____

A. Risk factors that impair social interaction
   1. Hearing and visual deficits
   2. Missing or diseased teeth
   3. Death of a spouse, other close relatives, and friends
   4. Retirement
   5. Lack of adequate transportation
   6. Living in a residential facility in which there are limited opportunities for solitude

B. Nursing interventions
   1. Encourage the client to discuss concerns about self-image, relationships, loneliness, or lack of privacy.
   2. Advise the client to correct obstacles to communication whenever possible (e.g., purchasing and wearing a hearing aid, having cataract surgery, undergoing restorative dentistry, having dentures repaired or replaced).
   3. Urge newly bereaved clients to verbalize their feelings and resume social activities at the appropriate time (e.g., by joining a widows' and widowers' support group).
   4. Encourage clients to prepare for retirement by making sound financial decisions, developing a circle of friends that is distinct from their friends at work, and becoming involved in personally fulfilling activities that offer opportunities for socialization.
   5. Assist clients who do not drive to identify affordable, dependable means of transportation.
   6. Allow clients who live in residential care facilities the option of spending some of their time alone in a quiet environment.

XII. Promoting appropriate sexuality

See text pages
_____

A. Risk factors to sexuality
   1. Factors that may disturb the self-image (e.g., wrinkled skin, graying and thinning hair, tooth loss or discoloration, decreased muscle tone, inflamed joints)
   2. Presence of chronic diseases that encourage preoccupation with health, cause continual discomfort, or restrict the number of positions that can be assumed

3. Need for increased physical stimulation to lubricate the vagina or achieve erection
4. Use of medications that can adversely affect libido, potency, orgasm, and ejaculation (e.g., sedatives, thiazide diuretics, tricyclic antidepressants, tranquilizers)
5. Disproportionate ratio of women to men among the elderly
6. Misconception that sexual activity is inappropriate during old age

B. Nursing interventions
1. Ensure that the sexual identity of elderly clients is respected by staff members, especially in long-term-care settings.
2. Assure clients that they can be sexually active as long as they are physically able.
3. Assist clients in overcoming physical, emotional, and environmental obstacles to sexuality.
4. Refer clients to a sex therapist or counselor if needed.
5. Provide privacy for the intimate encounters of clients who are institutionalized.
6. Offer suggestions about vaginal lubricants if inadequate lubrication causes painful intercourse.

See text pages

XIII. Promoting safety

A. Risk factors to safety
1. Decrease in intracellular fluid (increased risk of dehydration)
2. Lower basal metabolic rate and decrease in subcutaneous tissue (increased risk of hypothermia)
3. Decreased lung expansion, impairment of respiratory muscles and cough response, diseased teeth or gums, weakened gag reflex, increased urinary retention, increasingly alkaline vaginal secretions (increased risk of infection)
4. Impaired elimination of wastes from bloodstream, decreased glomerular filtration rate, decreased muscle strength, impaired physical mobility, delayed reaction time, impaired vision and hearing, distorted depth perception, decreased sensitivity to pain, impaired short-term memory, prevalence of polypharmacy

B. Nursing interventions
1. Teach the client self-assessment techniques that can be valuable means of detecting potentially serious conditions.
   a) Taking his/her pulse and temperature
   b) Listening to the lungs with a stethoscope
   c) Identifying possible adverse effects of drugs
   d) Detecting potentially significant changes in urine, feces, and sputum

2. Encourage the client to ingest the equivalent of 2 liters of fluid daily, half of which is water and may include fresh citrus fruits, ices, and Jell-O.

3. Urge the client to consume a well-balanced diet and help him/her to overcome common obstacles to good nutrition (see section VI,B of this chapter).

4. Advise the client to have regular evaluation of his/her vision and hearing and to wear prescribed eyeglasses or hearing aids.

5. Caution the client to avoid temperature fluctuations and extremes of heat and cold.

6. Advise the client that the baseline temperature of elderly individuals may drop significantly below 98.6°F, so it is possible to have a serious fever with a temperature of 99°F.

7. Caution the client to be alert to situations in which hypothermia can occur.

8. Warn clients against wearing clothing that can impair circulation in the extremities.

9. Explain to the client that because he/she is at increased risk of infection, exposure to persons with communicable infections should be avoided and immunizations should be kept up to date.

10. Caution the client to take prescribed medications as ordered, to be sure that all physicians and pharmacists are aware of each drug being taken, and never to take an over-the-counter drug before consulting the primary care physician.

11. Encourage the client to make use of written as well as oral instructions for drug administration and diagnostic test preparations.

12. Advise the client to eliminate structural and electrical hazards in the home and workplace; provide assistance, if necessary, in obtaining funds for needed repairs.

13. Instruct the client to prevent falls by eliminating improperly fitted canes or walkers, long robes, frayed carpeting, throw rugs, dimly lit rooms, and slippery floors and by using contrasting colors.

14. Encourage the client to clearly label medications, cleaning solutions, and other toxic materials.

15. Encourage the client to use transportation or escort services provided by local social service agencies.

16. Advise the client to check that shoes, orthotics, braces, canes, crutches, walkers, and wheelchairs are correctly sized and that, as appropriate, they are equipped with nonskid devices.

17. Urge the client to be particularly alert for criminals who prey on the elderly and to use caution when signing contracts and going out at night.

1. According to the free-radical theory of aging, the aging process may be retarded by:
   a. Hypothermia.
   b. Calorie restriction.
   c. Administration of antioxidant vitamins.
   d. Genetic engineering.

2. Which of the following statements represents accurate application of the activity theory of aging?
   a. Formal activity, such as paid employment, has a higher value than informal activity.
   b. Involvement in activities provided by a retirement community improves self-concept.
   c. Reduced energy levels in the elderly necessitate gradual withdrawal from activities.
   d. Lifetime habits determine the level of activities an older person will maintain.

3. According to Erikson, the developmental task of the elderly is:
   a. Retaining autonomy.
   b. Maintaining intimacy.
   c. Avoiding self-absorption.
   d. Establishing ego integrity.

4. Which of the following reflects Orem's theory of self-care?
   a. The nurse acts to help the client overcome limitations.
   b. The nurse predicts stressful events and prepares the client to cope with them.
   c. The nurse identifies a client's risk for illness and educates the client to change risk behaviors.
   d. The nurse prepares a written plan to guide client care activities.

5. Current dietary guidelines to promote cardiovascular health suggest that the elderly limit intake of fats to what percentage of total calories?
   a. 10%
   b. 30%

   c. 40%
   d. 50%

6. When teaching breathing exercises to the elderly client, the nurse needs to emphasize:
   a. The need to lie flat while performing the exercises.
   b. The importance of deep inhalation (sighing).
   c. The use of staged coughing to prevent excessive strain on respiratory muscles.
   d. The need for forced exhalation that lasts longer than inhalation.

7. Mrs. Farnum, age 90, reports that her limited income does not permit daily consumption of meat to provide dietary protein. Which of the following alternatives would provide complete protein at lower cost?
   a. Macaroni and cheese
   b. Cold cereal with milk
   c. Tomato soup and crackers
   d. Broccoli and rice

8. An appropriate suggestion for an elderly client who complains of itching would be:
   a. Bathe daily with Dove soap.
   b. Rub the itchy area with a terry cloth towel.
   c. Apply warm saline compresses to itchy areas.
   d. Use a room humidifier.

9. An elderly client complains of dribbling urine whenever she laughs or coughs. The appropriate nursing diagnosis to describe this problem is:
   a. Overflow incontinence.
   b. Functional incontinence.
   c. Stress incontinence.
   d. Urge incontinence.

10. To enhance the quality of a client's sleep, the nurse should advise the client to:
    a. Exercise 30 minutes before going to bed.
    b. Avoid over-the-counter analgesics within 2 hours of bedtime.

c. Develop a consistent bedtime routine.

d. Drink a glass of wine at bedtime.

11. Which of the following elderly clients is at greatest risk for social isolation?

a. A client who wears a hearing aid for deafness

b. A woman who recently moved from her own apartment to a retirement community

c. A man who lives in a rural area and cannot drive due to cataracts

d. A retired nurse who becomes a hospital volunteer

12. An 84-year-old woman reports vaginal pain with intercourse. Which suggestion by the nurse is most likely to help this client?

a. Apply a water-soluble lubricant to the vagina before intercourse.

b. Take a mild analgesic, such as Tylenol, prior to intercourse.

c. See your physician to be tested for a urinary tract infection.

d. Take a hot bath to relax your pelvic muscles before intercourse.

ANSWERS

1. **Correct answer is c.** Free radicals speed oxidation, which damages cell membranes. Vitamins A, C, and E are antioxidants, which limit this damage.

   a. Hypothermia applies to "biologic clock" theories; it delays the triggering of certain cell behaviors.

   b. Caloric restriction applies to the cross-link theory; it delays cross linking in rats.

   d. Genetic engineering applies to the immunologic theory. Immunoengineering approaches might control the development of autoimmune responses.

2. **Correct answer is b.** Activity theory postulates that continued involvement in activities promotes a positive self-concept.

a. Formal activity tends to be segregated by age and may therefore reinforce poor self-concept in the elderly.

c. The correspondence between reduced energy levels and withdrawal of the elderly from activities is consistent with disengagement theory.

d. The fact that lifetime habits have an effect on activities performed in old age is consistent with continuity (developmental) theory.

3. **Correct answer is d.** Accepting and finding meaning in one's life leads to ego integrity.

   a. Autonomy is the task of toddlers.

   b. Intimacy is the task of adolescence.

   c. Self-absorption reflects failure to achieve generativity, the task of middle age.

4. **Correct answer is a.** Orem's theory centers on promoting self-care whenever possible.

   b. Predicting stressful events reflects Roy's adaptation theory.

   c. Identifying risk for illness and education for change reflects wellness theory.

   d. Preparing a care plan is a part of the general nursing process and is not specific to a particular theory of nursing.

5. **Correct answer is b.** The American Heart Association guidelines suggest fats be limited to 30% of total calories. Most of this fat should be polyunsaturated.

   a. Although 10% might be desirable, it is unrealistic for most Americans.

   c and d. These percentages (40% and 50%) are higher than recommended and would increase the risk of cardiovascular disease.

6. **Correct answer is d.** The elderly commonly fail to exhale effectively. Breathing exercises must emphasize forced exhalation to compensate for this problem.

   a. Many elderly clients evidence some degree of orthopnea and cannot tolerate lying flat. A semi-Fowler's or erect position is a better choice.

b. Deep inhalation is important for the immobile or postoperative client to prevent atelectasis. It is not essential for all elderly clients.
c. Staged coughing is used for the immobile or postoperative client to prevent hypostatic pneumonia. It is not essential for all elderly clients.

7. **Correct answer is a.** The combination of cheese and pasta provides all the necessary amino acids for complete protein.

    b. Milk alone provides complete protein, but the serving size that is needed is larger than usually used on cereal. Also, cold cereals are often relatively expensive.
    c. A soup made with beans or lentils combined with bread or crackers would provide complete protein. Tomato soup does not.
    d. Rice and beans would provide complete protein. Broccoli with rice does not.

8. **Correct answer is d.** Dry skin often causes or exacerbates itching. Humidifying the air helps retain the skin's moisture.

    a. Use of a superfatted soap such as Dove would be appropriate, but daily bathing would deplete the skin's natural oils.
    b. Rubbing with a towel, like scratching, damages the skin and increases the itching.
    c. Compresses should be cold, not warm, because heat increases itching.

9. **Correct answer is c.** The client's condition is descriptive of stress incontinence.

    a. Overflow incontinence is manifested by frequent leakage of small amounts of urine without the bladder emptying.
    b. Functional incontinence occurs when the client is unaware of a need to void or cannot manage self-toileting.
    d. Urge incontinence occurs when the client cannot reach the toilet quickly enough when the urge to void is felt.

10. **Correct answer is c.** A consistent bedtime routine helps prepare the mind and body for sleep.

    a and **d.** Stimulating activities and substances close to bedtime can induce insomnia. Exercise, caffeine, alcohol, and smoking should be avoided.
    b. A mild analgesic at bedtime reduces the chances of being wakened by pain.

11. **Correct answer is c.** Because rural areas often lack public transportation, people living there who cannot drive are at high risk for social isolation.

    a. Sensory deficits are a risk factor, but correction of the deficit reduces the risk.
    b. Since most retirement communities provide planned activities for residents, this woman is less likely to be isolated in her new home than when she lived alone.
    d. Continuing contact with a familiar environment through volunteer activities reduces the retiree's risk of social isolation.

12. **Correct answer is a.** Reduced vaginal lubrication is a common age-related change. Dry vaginal mucosa can make intercourse very painful. A water-soluble lubricant will relieve the problem.

    b. The most likely cause of vaginal pain is decreased vaginal lubrication. Analgesics should not be used unless they are needed for another condition such as arthritis.
    c. Vaginal pain is not commonly a sign of urinary tract infection.
    d. Muscle tension or spasm might be relieved by a hot bath. However, decreased vaginal lubrication is the most likely cause of vaginal pain.

2

Physiologic and Psychosocial Assessments

I. **General characteristics associated with aging**
   A. Cells
   B. Body fluid
   C. Body fat
   D. Subcutaneous fat
   E. Body temperature
   F. Posture
   G. Tissue elasticity
   H. Body composition
   I. Senses

II. **Changes to body systems associated with normal aging process**
   A. Cardiovascular and peripheral vascular systems
   B. Respiratory system
   C. Gastrointestinal (GI) system
   D. Endocrine system
   E. Genitourinary and reproductive systems

   F. Musculoskeletal system
   G. Integumentary system
   H. Nervous system
   I. Immune system

III. **Cognitive and psychosocial characteristics associated with aging**
   A. Memory
   B. Intelligence
   C. Learning
   D. Personality

IV. **General principles of health assessment in the elderly client**
   A. Health history
   B. Physical assessment
   C. Functional assessment
   D. Psychosocial assessment

NURSING HIGHLIGHTS

1. In conducting the health assessment of an elderly person, the nurse should be alert to factors such as comfort, lack of privacy, background noise, fatigue, and sensory impairment, which may compromise the accuracy of the evaluation.
2. In conducting the physical assessment of an elderly client, the nurse must consider possible risks to the health of a frail older person, including examining rooms that are too cool, scales and examining tables from which the client may fall, and repeated changes in position, which may cause fatigue or postural hypotension.

GLOSSARY

fasciculation—a small local involuntary muscle contraction that is visible under the skin

fibrosis—increased fibrous tissue

hematopoiesis—production and development of blood cells

kyphosis—abnormal backward curvature of the spine

presbycusis—hearing loss that often develops with age

presbyopia—farsightedness that often develops with age

ptyalin—an enzyme found in saliva that converts starch into sugar

sclerosis—a condition characterized by hardening of tissue

vitiligo—skin disorder manifested by smooth white spots

ENHANCED OUTLINE

See text pages

_____

I. General characteristics associated with aging

A. Cells: gradual reduction in number

B. Body fluid: decrease in intracellular fluid (7%–10% less than younger adults), resulting in less total body fluid and increased chance of incidence of fluid and electrolyte imbalances

C. Body fat: atrophy of body fat, leading to deepening of hollows of intercostal and supraclavicular spaces, orbits, and axillae

D. Subcutaneous fat: decrease in subcutaneous fat, leading to reduction of skinfold thickness in forearm and on back of hands and decline in body's natural insulation

E. Body temperature: decrease in body's response to heat and cold; lowered ability to regulate temperature, leading to reduced ability to produce a fever to counter infection

F. Posture
  1. Loss of cartilage and thinning of vertebrae cause decrease in height.
  2. Vertebral osteoporosis, changes in cartilage, and muscle atrophy cause kyphosis.

G. Tissue elasticity: loss of elasticity due to degradation of elastin and collagen

H. Body composition: reduction in lean body mass and increase in fat mass

I. Senses
   1. Eyes
      a) General changes
         (1) Impaired reabsorption of intraocular fluid
         (2) Diminished corneal sensitivity
         (3) Decreased quantity and quality of tears causing increased incidence of infection, itching, and redness
      b) Vision
         (1) Presbyopia (see Chapter 11, section II,C,1,a)
         (2) Narrowing of visual field
         (3) Diminished responsiveness of pupil to light
         (4) Increased need for illumination but low tolerance for glare
         (5) Diminished perception of low-tone colors (e.g., blues, greens)
         (6) Distorted color perception due to yellowing of lens
         (7) Distorted depth perception
         (8) Decreased night vision
   2. Ears
      a) Hearing
         (1) Increasing presbycusis, beginning with high-frequency sounds (see Chapter 11, section II,C,2,a)
         (2) Increased keratin content of cerumen (earwax)
      b) Equilibrium: possible disturbances because of degeneration of vestibular structures, cochlea, organ of Corti, and stria vascularis
   3. Taste: diminished due to decreased number of functioning taste buds (sensitivity to sour, salty, and bitter tastes less affected than sensitivity to sweet tastes)
   4. Smell: diminished due to decreased number of sensory cells in nasal lining and reduced number of cells in olfactory bulb in brain
   5. Touch: reduced tactile sensation

II. Changes to body systems associated with normal aging process

A. Cardiovascular and peripheral vascular systems
   1. Vessels
      a) Aorta: dilation, elongation, and increased rigidity
      b) Blood vessels
         (1) Loss of elasticity, decreasing blood flow to organs (e.g., heart, kidneys) and causing decreased availability of oxygen, nutrients, antibodies, and immune cells
         (2) Narrowing of lumen size due to accumulation of fatty plaque and calcium deposits
         (3) Increase in peripheral vascular resistance (1%/year) due to arteriosclerosis
         (4) Increased vasomotor tone
         (5) Tortuous, engorged condition of vessels
   2. Heart
      a) Valves: thickening, calcification, and stiffening as a result of sclerosis and fibrosis

> See text pages
> _____

b) Output and volume
    (1) Overall slowing of heart rate
    (2) Loss of efficiency and contractile strength of heart muscle, leading to 30%–40% reduction of cardiac output (1%/year)
    (3) Decrease in stroke volume (0.7%/year)
    (4) Prolongation of isometric contraction phase and relaxation time of left ventricle
c) Tachycardia: takes longer for heart rate to elevate and to return to normal

3. Blood pressure
    a) Rise in systolic and diastolic blood pressure due to lack of elasticity, increased peripheral vascular resistance, and increased vasopressure lability
    b) Decreased baroreceptor activity

B. Respiratory system
  1. Musculoskeletal influences on respiratory system
    a) Rib cage: increased rigidity due to calcification of costal cartilage
    b) Chest: increased anterior-posterior chest diameter and some kyphosis, loss of water from vertebral discs
    c) Muscles: weakening and calcification of thoracic inspiratory and expiratory muscles
  2. Lungs
    a) General changes: loss of elasticity of lung tissues, reducing vital capacity; increase in residual volume with decrease in number of functioning alveoli, especially at lung base; decreased breath sounds; decreased ciliary action
    b) Alveoli: stretched and fewer in number, leading to lungs that are more rigid, with less recoil
    c) Expansion: decrease of lung expansion and insufficient basilar inflation
    d) Exhalation: less efficient exhalation, leading to increased residual volume; decreased ability to expel foreign or accumulated matter; diminished effectiveness of cough mechanism
    e) Respiratory infections: increased risk of respiratory infections

C. Gastrointestinal (GI) system
  1. Mouth and tongue: taste bud atrophy; decreased production of saliva and salivary ptyalin by as much as 66%
  2. Teeth: decreased dentin production, root pulp deterioration, gingival retraction, loss of alveolar-ridge bone density, possible tooth loss due to periodontal disease

3. Esophagus
   a) General changes: decreased motility, slight increase in dilation, delayed emptying time
   b) Sphincter: relaxation of lower sphincter resulting in increased incidence of reflux
4. Stomach
   a) General changes: decreased motility and hunger contractions and prolonged emptying time
   b) Gastric mucosa: atrophy of gastric mucosa
   c) Digestive enzymes: decreased production of digestive enzymes (lipase, pepsin, and hydrochloric acid)
5. Intestines
   a) General changes: some atrophy; fewer cells present on absorbing surfaces
   b) Absorption: decreased fat absorption and impaired absorption of dextrose, xylose, vitamin B_1 and vitamin B_{12}, calcium, and iron
   c) Muscles: decreased colonic peristaltic action; loss of tone in internal anal sphincter
   d) Neural impulses: dulling of impulses that sense signal to defecate
6. Liver: reduced size and storage capacity
7. Gallbladder: less efficient cholesterol stabilization and absorption; increased risk of gallstones
8. Pancreas
   a) General change: possible prolapse of entire gland
   b) Ducts: dilation and distention
   c) Enzymes: decreased production

D. Endocrine system
   1. Thyroid: decreased activity leading to lower basal metabolic rate
   2. Pituitary: decreased hormone production (adrenocorticotropic hormone, thyrotropin, follicle-stimulating hormone, luteinizing hormone, and luteotropic hormone)
   3. Gonads: gradual decline in secretion of testosterone, estrogen, and progesterone
   4. Pancreas: delayed and insufficient release of insulin, decreased sensitivity to circulating insulin, and reduced ability to metabolize glucose

E. Genitourinary and reproductive systems
   1. Kidneys
      a) General changes: decreased mass due to cortical loss, decline in tissue growth, decreased renal clearance, possible atrophy due to atherosclerosis
      b) Physiologic changes: decreased renal blood flow (53% drop due to reduced cardiac output) and decreased glomerular filtration rate (reduced by 50% between ages 40 and 90); decreased tubular function; decreased daily urinary creatinine excretion and creatinine clearance

2. Bladder
   a) General changes: decreased bladder innervation, weakened musculature and sphincter tone, decreased capacity
   b) Passage of urine: possible urine retention, delayed micturition reflex, possible stress incontinence
3. Male reproductive system: decreased testosterone production, decreased sperm count, some degree of benign prostatic hypertrophy in most elderly men (see Chapter 8, section II,C,4)
4. Female reproductive system
   a) Decreased estrogen production with menopause
   b) Breasts: Loss of firmness, atrophy
   c) Vulva: atrophy
   d) Labia: flattening
   e) Vagina: decreased vasculature, reduced secretions
   f) Cervix, uterus, fallopian tubes, and ovaries: atrophy and shrinking

F. Musculoskeletal system
   1. Muscle: decreased muscle mass, strength, and movements; muscle tremors
   2. Tendons: shrink and harden
   3. Reflexes: lost in abdomen; diminished in arms; retained in knees
   4. Bones
      a) General changes: reduction of bone mineralization and mass, gradual reabsorption of interior surface of long bones, slower production of new bone on outside surface
      b) Spine: thinning discs and shortening vertebrae, reducing length of spinal column; varying degrees of kyphosis
      c) Hips, wrists, and knees: slight flexion
      d) Joints: deterioration of cartilage surface; formation of points and spurs

G. Integumentary system
   1. Skin
      a) Sweat glands: diminished number and function of sweat glands, causing slight decrease in perspiration and less effective temperature regulation
      b) Thickness: flattening of dermal-epidermal junction, reduced thickness and vascularity of dermis, degeneration of elastin fibers
      c) Texture: increased fragility, dryness, and inflexibility of skin because of loss of subcutaneous fat, leading to wrinkles and sagging
      d) Susceptibility to injury: increased tendency to become irritated and break down
      e) Pigmentation: clustering of melanocytes

2. Hair
   a) General changes: graying and loss of hair
   b) Hair on chin and upper lip of women: coarse
   c) Hair in nostrils and ears of men: abundant
   d) Hair in the axillary and pubic areas, extremities, and trunk: decreased amounts
3. Nails: slower growth, increased brittleness and thickness, more yellow in color

H. Nervous system
   1. General change: reduction in number of nerve cells
   2. Cerebral blood flow and metabolism: reduced
   3. Nerve conduction velocity: lowered
   4. Kinesthetic sense: lessened

I. Immune system
   1. Overall function: decrease in natural antibodies, increase in autoantibodies, depressed immune response, decline in T-cell activity and production
   2. Response to vaccines: diminished responses to influenza, parainfluenza, pneumococcus, and tetanus vaccines
   3. Inflammatory defenses: decline in function

III. Cognitive and psychosocial characteristics associated with aging

See text pages
_____

A. Memory
   1. Immediate memory: rarely impaired significantly
   2. Recent memory
      a) Generally reduced
      b) Reduction sometimes intensified by physiologic factors (e.g., hypothermia) or psychosocial factors (e.g., the death of a spouse)
   3. Remote memory: rarely impaired significantly

B. Intelligence
   1. Basic intelligence: no change
   2. Verbal comprehension: no change
   3. Arithmetic skills: no change
   4. Crystallized intelligence (consists of the use of past learning and experiences for problem solving): no change
   5. Fluid intelligence (involves emotions, retention of nonintellectual information, creative capabilities, spatial perceptions, and aesthetic appreciation): apparent decline in some areas and in some aging people

Fluid intelligence

C. Learning
   1. Overall learning ability: not significantly affected by increasing age, although independent factors such as sensory deficits and illness can affect learning ability
   2. Perceptual motor tasks: increased difficulty due to slower reaction time and increase in cautious behavior

slower reaction time

3. Vigilance performance: decreased
4. Distractibility: increased
5. Performance of complex tasks or those associated with simultaneous performance: decreased ability, unless the individual has previous experience with the task

D. Personality
1. Basic personality traits: remain consistent over the years
2. Expression of personality: traits sometimes revealed more openly and honestly

IV. General principles of health assessment in the elderly client

See text pages

A. Health history
1. General guidelines
   a) Allow sufficient time.
   b) Use a comfortable, private, well-lit environment.
   c) Face the client at eye level.
   d) Use well-modulated speech tone and good diction.
   e) Use closed-ended questions, open-ended questions, and refocusing strategies as needed.
2. Basic information: name, address, telephone number, date of birth, gender, race, marital status, work status, living arrangements, notation about reliability of information
3. Presenting problem: the main symptom or cause of concern, phrased in the client's own language
4. History of current illness: summary and symptom analysis
5. Past health status: childhood illnesses, immunizations, allergies, major accidents, major adult illnesses, surgeries, hospitalizations, blood transfusions, obstetric history in women, exposure to environmental hazards, experience of living abroad or extensive foreign travel
6. Family history: general health statuses; ages at death; causes of death; presence of AIDS or related disorders, alcoholism, anemia, arthritis, cancer, cerebrovascular disease, developmental disability, diabetes mellitus, other endocrine disorders, headaches, heart disease, hypertension, psychiatric disorders, renal disorders, seizure disorders, tuberculosis
7. Personal habits: alcohol consumption; tobacco use; caffeine consumption; use of prescription, over-the-counter, and street drugs; use of nutritional supplements; frequency of physical examinations
8. Review of physiologic status: overall health, cardiovascular system, respiratory system, integumentary system, gastrointestinal system,

genitourinary system, breasts and axillae, musculoskeletal system, neurologic system, endocrine system, hematopoietic system

B. Physical assessment
1. General considerations
   a) Face the client at eye level; explain what the examination will involve and approximately how long it will last.
   b) Maintain the examining room at a temperature of 68°–75°F and ensure that the client's body is exposed for no longer than necessary because of the risk of hypothermia.
   c) Help the client to undress, if necessary, and provide a straight-back chair that can be used while removing shoes and underwear.
   d) Assist the client onto the scale and examining table, and do not leave the client unattended while sitting or lying on the examining table.
   e) Pad the examining table with a blanket if the client is thin; use pillows to aid breathing if necessary.
   f) Minimize the number of position changes that the client must make.
   g) Schedule 2 separate examination sessions if the client lacks the energy for a complete examination in 1 session.
   h) Take special care when examining the eyes, breasts, and genital region and when measuring blood pressure, as these may be areas of particular concern to the client.
2. Important areas for assessment in elderly clients
   a) General observation
      (1) Observe posture and gait; stooped posture and slow or altered gait may be present.
      (2) Listen for unusual sounds; wheezing during respiration may indicate illness.
      (3) Check for presence of involuntary movements (e.g., tremors).
      (4) Observe general cleanliness and grooming.
      (5) Check for unusual odors; breath or body odors may indicate illness.
      (6) Observe facial expression and affect.

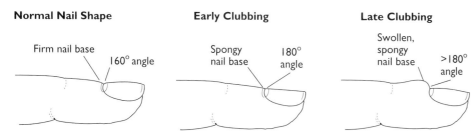

Figure 2–1
Stages of Clubbing

b) Skin
  (1) Observe color.
  (2) Take temperature.
  (3) Assess texture.
  (4) Check skin turgor, which may be decreased, with sagging, drooping, or wrinkling.
  (5) Check for presence of commonly occurring lesions or rashes (e.g., cherry angiomas, senile lentigines, seborrheic or actinic keratoses, cutaneous skin tags, vitiligo, purpuric lesions).
  (6) Inspect for presence of reddening at pressure areas, which may indicate tissue breakdown.
  (7) Inspect veins for varicosities.
c) Nails
  (1) Check for presence of fungus, cyanosis (bluish discoloration), and clubbing.
  (2) Check capillary refill time.
d) Head and neck
  (1) Check hair: color, texture, amount, distribution, cleanliness, presence of itching, lesions, or soreness.
  (2) Observe facial area.
    (a) Proportion and symmetry
    (b) Function of facial and trigeminal nerves during smiling, while pulling mouth side to side, while lifting lips to show teeth, and while resisting the health care provider's attempt to close the client's open mouth

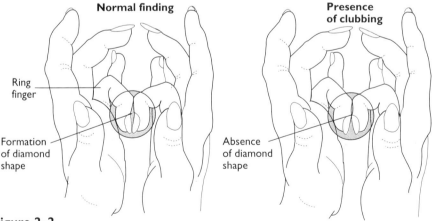

Figure 2–2
Testing for Clubbing: Schamrath Method

        (c) Presence of pain with movement of temporomandibular joint

    (3) Inspect eyes.
        (a) Alignment and symmetry
        (b) Presence of lid lag and inflammation
        (c) Color of sclera and conjunctiva
        (d) Pupils that are equal, round, and reactive to light and accommodation (PERRLA)
        (e) Presence of corneal irritation and opacities
        (f) Presence of lens opacities
        (g) Moisture and tearing

    (4) Assess ears.
        (a) Presence of tenderness, swelling, or nodules on auricle
        (b) Presence of cerumen, lesions, or discharge in auditory canal
        (c) Color and landmarks of tympanic membrane
        (d) Auditory acuity (using tuning fork)

    (5) Check nose.
        (a) Symmetry, shape, size, and color
        (b) Presence of masses
        (c) Presence of discharge or flaring of nares
        (d) Sense of smell (having the client identify strong odor)

    (6) Palpate frontal and maxillary sinuses for tenderness.

    (7) Assess mouth and oropharynx.
        (a) Presence of lesions on lips and in mouth
        (b) Condition of teeth for occlusion, number, color, and surface characteristics
        (c) Condition of gums
        (d) Fit of dentures
        (e) Swallowing and chewing abilities
        (f) Condition of mucous membranes
        (g) Function of gag reflex
        (h) Condition of buccal mucosa for color and texture and presence of lesions
        (i) Uvula midline
        (j) Tongue deviation
        (k) Presence of coating, redness, white patches, or lesions on tongue

    (8) Assess neck.
        (a) Range of motion
        (b) Function of spinal accessory nerve (ability to shrug shoulders)
        (c) Presence of enlargement or tenderness in lymph nodes
        (d) Presence of jugular vein distention

e) Thorax and lungs
    (1) Check symmetry of thorax.
    (2) Note respiratory rhythm, rate, and symmetry.

   (3) Test position and range of movement of diaphragm during inspiration and expiration.

   (4) Listen to breath sounds.

  f) Breasts and axillae

   (1) Check symmetry and contour.

   (2) Check for presence of masses or tenderness.

   (3) Observe nipples for discharge and inversion.

   (4) Assess for gynecomastia in males.

  g) Heart

   (1) Evaluate for presence of thrills or abnormal pulsations.

   (2) Assess rhythm and rate.

   (3) Check for presence of murmurs or other abnormal sounds.

   (4) Palpate point of maximal impulse (PMI).

  h) Peripheral vascular system

   (1) Measure blood pressure.

   (2) Assess coloring and warmth of extremities.

   (3) Check for presence of varicosities or ulceration.

  i) Abdomen

   (1) Assess contour (maximum height at level of umbilicus).

   (2) Determine size of liver by palpating upper and lower border.

   (3) Palpate for presence of masses or tenderness.

   (4) Auscultate bowel sounds.

  j) Musculoskeletal system

   (1) Assess body symmetry.

   (2) Assess muscle strength and atrophy.

   (3) Determine range of joint motion (e.g., flexion, extension, abduction, rotation).

   (4) Palpate joints for presence of tenderness, warmth, swelling, deformity, or crepitation (crackling).

  k) Nervous system

   (1) Test function of cranial nerves: control sense of smell, hearing, taste, corneal reflexes, facial muscles, peripheral vision, near vision, and movement of eyes.

   (2) Test motor nerve function: gait; equilibrium; coordination; hand grip; and presence of muscular atrophy, fasciculations, or involuntary movements.

   (3) Test sensory nerve function: perception of touch, temperature, pain, and vibration.

  l) Male genitalia

   (1) Inspect scrotum for symmetry, inflammation, edema, masses, or lesions.

      (2) Check rectum and anus for presence of inflammation, rash, lesions, hemorrhoids, masses; check stool for occult blood.

      (3) Check muscle tone of sphincter.

  m) Female genitalia and pelvis

      (1) Check vulva for inflammation, edema, tenderness, or masses.

      (2) Inspect vagina for color, odor, hydration status, lesions, mucosal bulging, excessive discharge, abnormal bleeding, and muscle tone.

      (3) Check for signs of prolapsed uterus.

      (4) Palpate size and consistency of ovaries.

      (5) Check rectum and anus for presence of inflammation, rash, lesions, hemorrhoids, masses.

      (6) Evaluate muscle tone of sphincter.

3. Age-related changes in common laboratory values

  a) Blood chemistry tests

      (1) Albumin: decreased because of smaller liver size and reduced blood flow and enzyme production

      (2) Alkaline phosphatase: increased, perhaps because of decreased liver function or poor vitamin D absorption

      (3) Blood urea nitrogen (BUN): increased because of decreased glomerular filtration rate and reduced renal tubular secretion

      (4) Creatinine: increased due to decreased kidney size

      (5) Calcium: slightly decreased perhaps due to inadequate intake

      (6) Fasting glucose: increased renal threshold for glucose

      (7) Glucose tolerance: deterioration; higher peak in 2 hours and slower decline to baseline

      (8) Potassium: slightly increased

      (9) Thyroxine (T_4): decreased because of slowed thyroid function

    (10) Uric acid: increased due, in women, to hormonal shifts in menopause

  b) Hematology tests

      (1) Hemoglobin: slightly decreased because of reduced hematopoiesis in men and women and decreased androgen levels in men

      (2) Hematocrit: slightly decreased because of reduced hematopoiesis

      (3) Leukocytes: decreased because of a decrease in T and B lymphocytes and reduced hematopoiesis

      (4) Sedimentation rate: slightly increased

  c) Creatinine clearance: must be calculated on the basis of decreased glomerular filtration rate

C. Functional assessment

  1. Purpose

    a) To assess performance in key functional areas to determine the client's ability to live independently

    b) To improve diagnostic evaluation

2. Areas of inquiry
   a) Work: the client's employment or occupation, including financial, interpersonal, or personal problems associated with retirement
   b) Sleep and rest: the amount and quality of sleep that the client gets in a typical day, including naps
   c) Recreation: the amount of time the client devotes to recreational activities and the type of activities in which he/she participates
   d) Stress reduction: the ways in which the client copes with stress, including the use of formal or informal stress-reduction techniques
   e) Nutritional practices
      (1) Description of a typical menu for 24 hours
      (2) Summary of normal fluid intake for 24 hours
      (3) The client's maximum and minimum weights during the past 5 years, past year, and past month
      (4) Any changes in appetite or food consumption patterns over the past year
      (5) Any problems experienced by the client that are associated with the selection, purchasing, transport, preparation, or eating of food
      (6) The amount of salt or sugar habitually added to food or beverages
   f) Exercise: the kind of exercise done and its frequency; any problems or discomfort experienced during exercise
   g) Activities of daily living (ADLs): activities related to personal hygiene and living independently
      (1) Dressing: the ability to handle buttons, zippers, and shoelaces and, for women, bras and garters
      (2) Grooming: the ability to brush the hair and teeth, shave, and cut the nails of the hands and feet
      (3) Bathing: the ability to prepare bath water, get into or out of the bath or shower, and wash all parts of the body
      (4) Toileting: the ability to access the toilet and clean the body after using the toilet
      (5) Eating: the ability to cut food, handle utensils, and put food in the mouth; the ability to chew and swallow without choking
      (6) Mobility: the ability to walk throughout the house, get into and out of bed, lower to and rise from a chair, climb stairs, and reach for items in cupboards
   h) Instrumental activities of daily living (IADLs): the more difficult activities related to home management

KATZ INDEX OF ACTIVITIES OF DAILY LIVING
EVALUATION FORM

Name _____ Date of Evaluation _____

Independence means without supervision, direction, or active personal assistance, except as specifically noted below. This is based on actual status and not ability. A patient who refuses to perform a function is considered as not performing the function, even though he or she is deemed able.

For each area of functioning listed below, circle description that applies (the word "assistance" means supervision, direction, or personal assistance).

Bathing—either sponge bath, tub bath, or shower

Receives no assistance (gets in and out of tub by self if tub is usual means of bathing)	Receives assistance in bathing only one part of body (such as back or a leg)	Receives assistance in bathing more than one part of body (or does not bathe self)

Dressing—gets clothes from drawers; puts on clothes, including underclothes, outer garments; manages fasteners (including braces, if worn)

Gets clothes and gets completely dressed without assistance	Gets clothes and gets dressed without assistance except for tying shoes	Receives assistance in getting clothes or in getting dressed or stays partly or completely undressed

Toileting—going to the "toilet room" for bowel and urine elimination; cleaning self after elimination and arranging clothes

Goes to "toilet room," cleans self, and arranges clothes without assistance (may use object for support such as cane, walker, or wheelchair and may manage night bedpan or commode, emptying same in morning)	Receives assistance in going to "toilet room" or in cleaning self or in arranging clothes after elimination or in use of night bedpan or commode	Does not go to room termed "toilet" for the elimination process

Transfer

Moves in and out of bed and in and out of chair without assistance (may use objects for support such as cane or walker)	Moves in or out of bed with assistance	Does not get out of bed

Continence

Controls urination and bowel movement completely by self	Has occasional "accidents"	Supervision helps keep urine or bowel control; catheter is used or is incontinent

Feeding

Feeds self without assistance	Feeds self except for getting assistance in cutting meat or buttering bread	Receives assistance in feeding or is fed partly or completely by tubes or intravenous fluids

SOURCE: Katz, S., et al. 1963. Studies of illness in the aged: The index of ADL: A standardized measure of biological and psychological function. *JAMA* 185:914–919. Copyright © 1963, American Medical Association.

Figure 2-3
Katz Index of Activities of Daily Living Evaluation Form

         (1) Telephone: the ability to read telephone numbers, dial the phone or press the appropriate buttons, hear the phone ring, and hear conversation over the phone

         (2) Housekeeping: the abilities to clean the house, make the bed, wash dishes, and take out garbage

         (3) Food preparation: the ability to plan, prepare, and serve appropriate meals

         (4) Laundry: the ability to wash and dry one's own clothing

         (5) Money management: the ability to establish and follow a budget, write checks or money orders, and use bills and coins

         (6) Medication management: the ability to take prescribed medications in the right dose at the right time and follow any instructions about dietary or other restrictions

         (7) Access to transportation: the ability to use a car or public transportation to get to the doctor, the supermarket, or other chosen destinations

   3. Formal tools often used in the functional assessment of the elderly client

      a) Barthel Index: an evaluation, based on a 1–100 scale, of a client's self-care abilities and degree of mobility

      b) Functional Independence Measure: an evaluation of a client's self-care abilities, sphincter control, mobility, locomotion, communication, and social cognition

      c) Katz Index of Activities of Daily Living Evaluation Form: an inventory of a client's degree of independence in bathing, dressing, toileting, transfer out of bed, continence, and feeding

      d) Scale for Instrumental Activities of Daily Living: an evaluation used to determine the client's ability to use the telephone, go shopping, prepare food, keep house, do laundry, travel independently, take own medication, and handle finances

D. Psychosocial assessment

   1. For use in mental status or psychologic assessment of the elderly client

   2. General guidelines

      a) Ensure that the physical environment is quiet, private, and comfortable; if possible, the place should be familiar to the client.

      b) Introduce yourself at the beginning of the interview and describe the kind of information that will be sought.

      c) Determine as quickly as possible whether sensory deficits are present and adapt questioning accordingly.

      d) Try to reduce the client's initial anxiety by beginning the interview with less personal subjects.

e) Observe the client for signs of fatigue and abbreviate the interview or schedule another session if he/she is excessively tired.

f) Summarize the content of the interview at the end of the session.

3. Usual components of the assessment

a) General appearance: hygiene; grooming; absence of odor; age-appropriate clothing, use of cosmetics, and hairstyle; normal posture (allowing for age-related changes); appropriate facial expression and eye contact

---

Mini-Mental State Examination

	Maximum score	Score
Orientation		
What is the (year) (season) (date) (day) (month)?	5	(_____)
Where are we (state) (county) (town) (hospital) (floor)?	5	(_____)
Registration		
Name 3 objects: I second to say each. Then ask the patient all 3 after you have said them. Give 1 point for each correct answer. Then repeat them until he learns all 3. Count trials and record. _____ Trials	3	(_____)
Attention and calculation		
Serial 7's. 1 point for each correct. Stop after 5 answers. Alternatively spell "world" backwards.	5	(_____)
Recall		
Ask for the 3 objects repeated above. Give 1 point for each correct.	3	(_____)
Language		
Name a pencil and a watch. (2 points)	9	(_____)
Repeat the following: "No ifs, ands, or buts." (1 point)		
Follow a 3-stage comment: "Take a paper in your right hand, fold it in half, and put it on the floor." (3 points)		
Read and obey the following: Close your eyes. (1 point) Write a sentence. (1 point) Copy design. (1 point)		
TOTAL SCORE		_____

Assess level of consciousness along a continuum

Alert	Drowsy	Stupor	Coma

SOURCE: Reprinted from Folstein, M. F., S. E. Folstein, and P. R. McHugh. 1975. The Mini-Mental State Examination. *Journal of Psychiatric Research* 12:189–198. Copyright © 1975 by Pergamon Press Ltd. Reprinted by permission of Pergamon Press Ltd., an imprint of Elsevier Science Ltd.

Figure 2–4
Mini-Mental State Examination

       b) Psychomotor behavior: rate of movement, gait, coordination, appropriateness of movements, absence of involuntary movements, appropriate handshake

       c) Level of consciousness: responsive to stimuli; appropriate orientation to time, place, and person

       d) Affect: appropriate to the situation, congruency of verbal and nonverbal language

       e) Ability to pay attention: appropriate responses to questions, train of thought maintained

       f) Speech: appropriate rate, volume, clarity, and amount; use of vocabulary that is appropriate to educational and socioeconomic level

       g) Understanding: comprehension of the interviewer's questions and comments

       h) Thought patterns: appropriate flow of thought and transitions

       i) General knowledge: basic awareness of current events and bodily processes

       j) Judgment: appropriate response to illness and to interview situation

       k) Impulse control: cooperates with the interviewer and responds appropriately to questions

  4. Common tools used in the psychosocial assessment of the elderly client

       a) Mini-Mental State Examination (MMSE): test of cognitive ability that evaluates the client's orientation, attention, and recall and ability to understand and use language and reproduce a geometric diagram

       b) Short Portable Mental Status Questionnaire (SPMSQ): test of cognitive ability that measures orientation, knowledge of current events, and ability to perform a simple arithmetic calculation

       c) The Set Test: test of cognitive ability in which the client is asked to name as many colors, animals, fruits, and towns as possible, up to a maximum of 10 per category

       d) Blessed Dementia Rating Scale: evaluation of the client's ability to perform everyday activities (e.g., handling small sums of money, finding the way around familiar streets, eating, dressing, toileting)

       e) Geriatric Depression Scale or Mood Assessment Scale: used to screen for and determine severity of depression

       f) Michigan Alcoholism Screening Test (MAST): diagnostic test in which the client is asked questions about the effect that drinking has or has had on his/her everyday life

g) The Burden Interview: used to estimate the degree of stress that the caregiver of a spouse is experiencing

h) Nowotny Hope Scale: used to measure the client's capacities for dealing constructively with a stressful event

CHAPTER 2 · REVIEW QUESTIONS

1. Which of the following age-related pulmonary changes is expected in healthy elderly adults?
   a. Decreased lung size
   b. Hyperinflation of the alveoli at the bases
   c. Reduced total lung capacity
   d. Decreased effectiveness of cough mechanism

2. The nurse should monitor the elderly client for signs of deficiency of:
   a. Vitamin B_{12}.
   b. Vitamin C.
   c. Glucose.
   d. Potassium.

3. Age-related changes in the pancreas are likely to produce which of the following changes in laboratory test values in the elderly client?
   a. Decreased fasting blood sugar
   b. Lower peak glucose level on glucose tolerance test
   c. Prolonged time to return to baseline on glucose tolerance test
   d. Higher peak with a rapid drop to baseline on glucose tolerance test

4. When performing health assessment of the elderly client, the nurse should consider which of the following abnormal?
   a. Flattened labia
   b. Dribbling of urine
   c. Elevated blood urea nitrogen (BUN)
   d. Decreased amount of urine passed with each voiding

5. When testing the healthy elderly client's reflexes, the nurse would expect to find which of the following?
   a. Increased abdominal reflexes
   b. Increased Achilles tendon reflex
   c. Diminished brachial reflex
   d. Diminished knee jerk reflex

6. Which of the following integumentary changes would be considered abnormal in an elderly client?
   a. Poor skin turgor on the hand or forearm
   b. Thick, yellow toenails
   c. Decreased perspiration in the axillary area
   d. Absence of hair on the feet and ankles

7. When evaluating memory in an elderly person, the nurse is most likely to observe abnormalities with which test?
   a. Recall of a series of digits in 2–3 minutes
   b. Naming family members
   c. Describing the previous night's dinner
   d. Recalling events from childhood

8. In which aspect of intelligence would a normal age-related decline be expected?
   a. Creativity
   b. Problem solving
   c. Mathematical calculations
   d. Verbal comprehension

9. When an elderly client complains of chronic fatigue, it is especially important for the nurse to assess:
   a. Dietary habits.
   b. Condition of the integument.
   c. Sensory function.
   d. Results of blood urea nitrogen (BUN) and creatinine tests.

10. The nurse should expect to find that, because of changes associated with the normal aging process, an elderly client's hematocrit values will be:
    a. Slightly increased.
    b. Greatly increased.

c. Slightly decreased.

d. Greatly decreased.

11. Assessment of instrumental activities of daily living (IADLs) would include evaluation of:

a. Grooming.

b. Telephone use.

c. Stress management.

d. Recreational activities.

12. When performing a psychosocial assessment of an elderly client, the nurse should:

a. Take the client to a neutral environment such as a conference room.

b. Permit the client to direct the content of the interview to the client's most pressing concerns.

c. Divide the interview into 2 sessions to reduce fatigue if the client seems tired.

d. Include a family member in the interview to validate information obtained from the client.

ANSWERS

1. **Correct answer is d.** Decreased inflation of lung bases and reduced ciliary function result in decreased effectiveness of the cough mechanism.

a. Lung size does not decrease, although the lungs become more rigid so they do not expand or recoil as effectively.

b. Inflation of the lung bases decreases with incomplete lung expansion. At the same time lung rigidity may result in increased inflation of the apices.

c. Total lung capacity does not change. However, increased residual capacity causes a decrease in vital capacity.

2. **Correct answer is a.** Reduced secretion of hydrochloric acid (intrinsic factor) in the elderly impairs the absorption of vitamin B_{12}.

The elderly on limited incomes may not eat the animal protein foods that are good sources of vitamin B_{12} since they tend to be expensive. Chewing problems may make ingestion of these foods difficult.

b, c, and **d.** Vitamin C, glucose, and potassium are all found in many foods and beverages and are less likely to be deficient in the diet of the elderly. Absorption of these substances is not normally impaired.

3. **Correct answer is c.** The elderly commonly have a prolonged return to baseline on glucose tolerance tests.

a. Fasting blood sugar is commonly increased.

b. Peak glucose level on glucose tolerance tests is normally higher in the elderly than in younger adults.

d. The peak glucose level is higher, but the return to baseline is prolonged.

4. **Correct answer is b.** Incontinence should not be considered normal. Dribbling may indicate urine retention with overflow incontinence due to prostatic hypertrophy or correctable structural problems such as cystocele.

a. Flattening of the labia is a common age-related change.

c. Some elevation of BUN is common. As nephrons are lost due to age, the kidneys become less efficient at excreting nitrogen wastes.

d. Bladder capacity often decreases with age, resulting in increased frequency of voiding with smaller amounts voided each time. Also, sphincter strength decreases, so that less urine can be stored before voiding.

5. **Correct answer is c.** The brachial reflexes are usually diminished in the elderly.

a and **b.** Both abdominal and Achilles reflexes are diminished in the elderly. Abdominal reflexes may be absent.

d. Knee jerk reflex is normally unchanged in the elderly.

6. **Correct answer is d.** Absence of hair is an indication of impaired circulation. This would be abnormal, indicating peripheral vascular disease.

   a. Normal age-related decrease in subcutaneous fat causes poor skin turgor as well as wrinkles and sagging.
   b. The nails become thicker, yellowed, and brittle with age.
   c. Sweat glands decrease in number and function with age, causing a slight decrease in perspiration in the elderly.

7. **Correct answer is c.** Describing the previous evening's meal tests recent memory, which is most likely to be impaired in the elderly.

   a. Recalling a series of numbers in 2–3 minutes tests immediate memory, which is rarely impaired significantly with normal aging.
   b. Recalling names of family members would be lost only in the most severe stages of dementia.
   d. Recalling childhood events tests remote memory, which is rarely impaired significantly with normal aging.

8. **Correct answer is a.** Creativity reflects fluid intelligence, the only area in which an apparent decline occurs with age.

   b. Problem solving reflects crystallized intelligence, which does not change with aging.
   c and **d.** Verbal comprehension and math skills do not change with normal aging.

9. **Correct answer is a.** Nutritional deficits are a common cause of fatigue.

   b, c, and **d.** These assessments do not directly address the most likely causes of fatigue. Muscle tone, cardiovascular and respiratory status, and drug history are more essential. Important laboratory studies include complete blood count (CBC), glucose, thyroid function, and electrolyte levels.

10. **Correct answer is c.** Reduced hematopoiesis, which is part of the normal aging process, results in a slight decrease in hematocrit in the elderly.

    a and **b.** Increased hematocrit often indicates dehydration, which would be abnormal.
    d. Greatly decreased hematocrit may reflect anemia, an abnormality which impairs oxygenation and exacerbates cardiac and respiratory problems.

11. **Correct answer is b.** Instrumental activities of daily living (IADLs) are the activities related to home management and include telephoning, housekeeping, transportation, and the management of finances.

    a. Grooming is a basic activity of daily living (ADL) that is assessed with other activities related to personal hygiene such as bathing and dressing.
    c and **d.** Stress management and recreation are important but are not IADLs.

12. **Correct answer is c.** Attention span may be shorter in the elderly client. Long interviews can be fatiguing to the elderly. Dividing the interview into multiple sessions can improve attention and responsiveness by decreasing fatigue.

    a. Elderly clients may be more comfortable, and therefore more open, in a familiar environment. Psychosocial assessment should occur in the client's home or own room.
    b. While it is appropriate to use open-ended questions that allow the client to express concerns, the nurse must direct the content of the interview to be sure that all important information is covered.
    d. Privacy is important. Unless the elderly person is seriously impaired, he/she can provide accurate information. The presence of a family member may inhibit open communication.

3

Drug Use and Abuse and the Elderly Client

NURSING HIGHLIGHTS

1. The nurse should be alert for drug-related problems among the elderly because, due to changes in pharmacokinetics and pharmacodynamics, older people are more likely than younger adults to experience adverse reactions, drug-drug interactions, and drug-food interactions.
2. The nurse should be attentive to subtle signs of alcohol abuse in older adults. Age-related changes can exaggerate adverse effects of drug and alcohol combinations, resulting in life-threatening problems.
3. The nurse should be aware that the client with an alcohol abuse problem and the members of his/her family may underestimate or conceal the problem.

GLOSSARY

absorption—the process by which medication introduced into the body enters the general circulation

distribution—transport of a drug through the body

metabolism—the enzymatic alteration of a drug molecule (also called biotransformation)

pharmacodynamics—the study of drug effects at the receptor level

pharmacokinetics—the absorption, distribution, metabolism, and excretion of drugs

polypharmacy—the use of more than 1 drug at a time for 1 or more health problems, with drugs sometimes being prescribed by more than 1 physician

ENHANCED OUTLINE

See text pages
_____

I. Pharmacokinetics in the elderly

A. Absorption
1. Factors that can alter drug absorption in older clients
   a) Age-related changes: decreased gastric acidity, reduced gastrointestinal blood flow and motility, prolonged gastric emptying time, decrease in the number of absorbing cells, decrease in the number of mucus-secreting cells
   b) Conditions: diabetes mellitus and hypokalemia (increased absorption), congestive heart failure (decreased absorption)
2. Means of increasing drug absorption
   a) Perform measures that increase blood flow at the absorption site (e.g., helping the client exercise, applying heat, giving a massage) unless contraindicated by the client's condition.
   b) Prevent fluid volume deficit, hypotension, and hypothermia.
   c) Monitor drug-drug and drug-food interactions.
   d) For each client, administer the drug by the most efficient route available.
   e) Control the client's pain, and reduce emotional stress.

B. Distribution
1. Factors that may affect drug distribution in older clients
   a) Age-related changes: increase in adipose tissue, reduced total body mass, reduction in lean body mass, decrease in total body water, reduced serum albumin, decreased cardiac output
   b) Drug solubility and concentration: prolonged effect of fat-soluble drugs (e.g., diazepam), decreased effect of highly water-soluble

drugs, increased risk of toxicity of highly protein-bound drugs (e.g., amitriptyline, chlorpromazine, digitoxin, furosemide, phenytoin, warfarin)

    c) Conditions: dehydration, hypoalbuminemia, poor nutrition, prolonged bed rest, electrolyte imbalances

  2. Means of increasing drug distribution

    a) Avoid, when possible, the coadministration of 2 or more highly protein-bound drugs.

    b) Maintain adequate fluid volume and normal electrolyte balance.

    c) Adjust drug dosages to compensate for increased adipose tissue, decreased lean tissue, and/or hypoalbuminemia.

C. Metabolism and excretion

  1. Factors that can alter metabolism and excretion in older clients

    a) Age-related changes

      (1) Reduced kidney efficiency (especially lower glomerular filtration rate), causing drugs to remain in the body for a longer time and increasing the risk of adverse reactions, including toxicity

      (2) Decreased size and function of the liver

        (a) Impairs the formation of prothrombin, albumin, and vitamins A, B_{12}, and D

        (b) Impairs the production of enzymes needed for metabolism of some drugs

        (c) Delays the detoxification and conjugation of drugs

    b) Conditions: dehydration, hyperthermia, liver disease, cardiovascular disease, renal disease, congestive heart failure, immobility

  2. Means of increasing metabolism and excretion

    a) Maintain adequate hydration and normal body temperature.

    b) Encourage the client to exercise to tolerance.

    c) Carefully monitor creatinine clearance and serum creatinine levels.

    d) Carefully monitor drugs that depend on hepatic blood flow to metabolize (e.g., propranolol), drugs that interfere with hepatic enzyme metabolism (e.g., cimetidine), and nephrotoxic drugs (e.g., gentamicin, carbenicillin).

II. Adverse drug reactions experienced by the elderly

See text pages

A. Causes of adverse reactions

  1. Normal age-related physiologic changes that affect pharmacokinetics and pharmacodynamics (see Chapter 2, sections I and II)

  2. Acute disease or chronic condition

  3. Polypharmacy

    a) Causes

      (1) Older clients often have more than 1 acute or chronic health problem or a chronic disease that is treated with more than 1 drug.

(2) Multiple physicians may be prescribing drugs at the same time.

(3) The elderly tend to have more faith in pharmacotherapy than other treatment methods.

(4) The elderly may self-medicate with over-the-counter (OTC) drugs in addition to using prescription drugs.

(5) An adverse reaction to 1 drug may be misinterpreted as a new condition for which a second drug is prescribed.

b) Common combinations of drugs taken by the elderly

(1) Diuretics, tranquilizers, and potassium

(2) Vitamins, minerals, and laxatives

(3) Digitalis preparations with diuretics

(4) Tranquilizers, sedatives, and gastrointestinal (GI) preparations

(5) GI preparations with tranquilizers, diuretics, and vitamins

4. Poor compliance

a) Perceived lack of efficacy, disagreeable side effects, or the resolution of symptoms (see Nurse Alert, "Behaviors Associated with Poor Compliance with Drug Regimens")

b) Concern about the cost of a drug, causing the client to postpone filling a prescription or to take the drug less often than prescribed

c) Incomplete understanding of the regimen

(1) Directions are given too quickly or when the client is uncomfortable or distressed, medical jargon is used, or the primary language of the client is not used.

(2) The client is embarrassed to mention a lack of understanding due to a hearing problem or poor reading ability.

d) Forgetfulness

e) Confusion related to multiple drug regimens

5. Narrow therapeutic indices (i.e., closeness of therapeutic and toxic levels) of many drugs taken by elderly clients (e.g., anticoagulants, antihypertensives, antidepressants, digitalis glycosides)

B. Main drugs causing adverse reactions in the elderly (some side effects may occur in all clients but are exacerbated in elderly clients; drug reactions that are common or of particular concern in the elderly are italicized)

1. Analgesics

a) Aspirin: GI bleeding, peptic ulcer, central nervous system (CNS) dysfunction

b) Codeine: constipation, drowsiness

c) Meperidine: *delirium,* dizziness, hypotension, impaired mental and physical functioning

Behaviors Associated with Poor Compliance with Drug Regimens

Noncompliance is a major cause of treatment failure and can be life-threatening for elderly clients. Be aware of behaviors associated with poor compliance.

- Neglecting to have a prescription filled
- Ordering drugs by mail or telephone, thus missing instructions for administration
- Failing to open childproof caps on medication containers
- Taking drugs at the wrong time
- Taking double doses to compensate for a missed dose
- Taking prescribed and OTC drugs without an understanding of potentially serious interactions
- Failing to understand that OTC preparations such as vitamins and antacids are drugs that can have serious adverse effects and cause dangerous interactions
- Improperly storing medications where they may be damaged by excess heat, humidity, or light
- Discontinuing medications once symptoms are relieved, despite instruction to continue for control of a chronic condition
- Stockpiling out-of-date drugs for future use
- Swapping medications with others who have similar symptoms

    d) Morphine sulfate: decreased heartbeat and peristalsis, disorientation, euphoria, increased sphincter muscle tone, respiratory depression

2. Antacids: diarrhea (with magnesium hydroxide); hypernatremia, metabolic alkalosis (with sodium bicarbonate); hypercalcemia (with calcium carbonate); renal disorders (with calcium antacids); constipation (with aluminum hydroxide)

3. Antianxiety drugs: bladder control problems, CNS depression, confusion, constipation, dizziness, double vision, drowsiness, dry mouth, GI problems, immunologic impairment, photosensitivity, slurred speech, unsteadiness (see also Chapter 12, sections V,A and V,C)

4. Anticoagulants: internal bleeding; osteoporosis, spontaneous fractures (with heparin)

5. Anticonvulsants: GI irritation; ataxia, coma, delirium, disorientation, emotional disturbance (with phenobarbital); visual hallucinations, anemia (with primidone); gingival hyperplasia (with phenytoin)

6. Antidepressants: arrhthymias, anticholinergic effects (e.g., constipation, urinary retention, delirium, blurred vision), orthostatic hypotension, psychosis, sedation, tremors (see also Chapter 12, sections V,A and V,C)

7. Antidiabetic drugs (chlorpropamide more dangerous than tolbutamide): hypoglycemia, cardiovascular morbidity

8. Antihypertensive agents: drowsiness, orthostatic hypotension
   a) Calcium channel blockers: *constipation, edema,* flushing, headache, palpitations, tachycardia
   b) Methyldopa: *altered cognition, anemia, depression, edema,* angina pectoris, hepatitis, reversible liver damage
   c) Propranolol and nadolol: *fatigue, feeling of coldness, heart failure, insomnia,* angina when stopped suddenly, bradycardia, diarrhea, dizziness, hallucinations, nightmares, psychotic disturbances
9. Anti-infectives: *bleeding, bacterial superinfection with resulting severe diarrhea;* depressed plasma prothrombin activity (with tetracycline); hepatotoxicity (with antituberculars); hypokalemia (with carbenicillin); nephrotoxicity, ototoxicity (with aminoglycosides)
10. Anti-inflammatory drugs: GI disorders
    a) Colchicine: anorexia, confusion, convulsions, diarrhea, muscle weakness, peripheral neuritis
    b) Corticosteroids: bone demineralization, fluid retention, immune system impairment, sodium retention
    c) Nonsteroidal anti-inflammatory drugs (NSAIDs): sodium and fluid retention, GI distress or bleeding, renal failure, confusion
11. Antiparkinson drugs: involuntary movements, restlessness, nightmares, hallucinations, psychosis (with levodopa and carbidopa/levodopa); dizziness, ataxia, insomnia, hypotension (with amantadine)
12. Antipsychotic agents (also called major tranquilizers): anticholinergic symptoms (e.g., dry mouth, constipation, blurred vision, confusion, fever, agitation), extrapyramidal symptoms (e.g., unusual movements of the mouth and tongue, abnormal limb movements and gait, rigidity of muscles in neck and trunk), orthostatic hypotension, sedation (see also Chapter 12, sections V,B and V,C)
13. Cardiotonics: anorexia with weight loss, dizziness, GI disturbances, visual disturbances; *confusion* (with digitalis)
14. Diuretics: blood disorders, diarrhea, fluid and electrolyte imbalances (especially hypokalemia), headache, orthostatic hypotension, photosensitivity, tinnitus, urge incontinence; increased or decreased blood glucose levels, elevated serum lipids (with thiazides); ototoxicity (with loop diuretics)
15. Laxatives: chronic constipation, excessive fluid loss, intestinal cramps
16. Nitrates: *cranial throbbing, dizziness, orthostatic hypotension, increased intraocular pressure,* blurred vision, confusion, decreased respiration, dizziness, flushing, irregular and rapid pulse, muscle weakness
17. Sedatives and hypnotics (includes minor tranquilizers): confusion, disorientation, dizziness, drowsiness, hypotension, impaired coordination, incontinence, irritability

III. Drug interactions experienced by the elderly

See text pages

A. Major drug-drug interactions by therapeutic class

   1. Analgesics
      a) Aspirin: increased effects of oral anticoagulants, oral antidiabetics, corticosteroids, penicillins, phenytoin; decreased effects of probenecid, spironolactone, sulfinpyrazone; effects of aspirin increased by vitamin C; effects of aspirin decreased by antacids, phenobarbital, propranolol, reserpine
      b) Acetaminophen: effects decreased by phenobarbital; risk of toxicity increased by high doses (>500 mg/day) of vitamin C
      c) Narcotic analgesics: increased effects of antidepressants, sedatives, tranquilizers, other analgesics; effects of narcotics increased by antidepressants, phenothiazines
      d) Meperidine: decreased effects of antiglaucoma eyedrops; effects of meperidine increased by nitrates

   2. Antacids
      a) Most antacids: decreased effects of barbiturates, chlorpromazine, digoxin, iron, isoniazid, nitrofurantoin, oral anticoagulants, penicillins, phenytoin, salicylates, sulfonamides, tetracycline, vitamins A and C
      b) Aluminum hydroxide: increased effects of meperidine, pseudoephedrine
      c) Magnesium hydroxide: increased effects of dicumarol

   3. Antianxiety drugs: increased effects of anticonvulsants, antihypertensives, oral anticoagulants, other central nervous system (CNS) depressants; effects of antianxiety drugs increased by tricyclic antidepressants

   4. Anticoagulants
      a) Increased effects of hypoglycemic agents, phenytoin
      b) Decreased effects of cholestyramine
      c) Effects of anticoagulants increased by alcohol, antibiotics, chloral hydrate, chlorpromazine, cimetidine, colchicine, ethacrynic acid, phenylbutazone, phenytoin, probenecid, reserpine, salicylates, steroids, thyroxine, tolbutamide, tricyclic antidepressants
      d) Effects of anticoagulants decreased by antacids, barbiturates, carbamazepine, chlorpromazine, cholestyramine, rifampin, vitamins C and K

   5. Anticonvulsants
      a) Increased effects of analgesics, antihistamines, propranolol, sedatives, tranquilizers
      b) Decreased effects of cortisone
      c) Effects of anticonvulsants increased by isoniazid; by coumarin anticoagulants, effects of phenytoin increased and effects of phenobarbital decreased

   6. Antidepressants
      a) Increased effects of anticoagulants, antihistamines, atropine, levodopa, narcotics, sedatives, tranquilizers

b) Decreased effects of antihypertensives, clonidine, phenytoin

c) Effects of antidepressants increased by alcohol, thiazide diuretics

7. Antidiabetic drugs

   a) Effects of antidiabetic drugs increased by alcohol, isoniazid, oral anticoagulants, phenylbutazone, salicylates, sulfinpyrazone

   b) Effects of antidiabetic drugs decreased by chlorpromazine, corticosteroids, furosemide, phenytoin, thiazides, thyroid preparations

8. Antihypertensive agents

   a) Increased effects of barbiturates, insulin, oral antidiabetics, sedatives, thiazides

   b) Propranolol: decreased effects of antihistamines, anti-inflammatory drugs

   c) Effects of antihypertensive agents increased by phenytoin

   d) Effects of antihypertensive agents decreased by amphetamines, antihistamines, tricyclic antidepressants

9. Anti-infectives

   a) Effects of most antibiotics increased by probenecid

   b) Ampicillin and carbenicillin: effects decreased by antacids, chloramphenicol, erythromycin, tetracycline

   c) Doxycycline: effects decreased by alcohol, antacids, iron, laxatives, phenobarbital

   d) Penicillins: decreased effects of other protein-bound drugs; effects of penicillin decreased by other protein-bound drugs

   e) Sulfisoxazole: increased effects of alcohol, oral anticoagulants, oral antidiabetics, methotrexate, phenytoin; effects of sulfisoxazole increased by aspirin, oxyphenbutazone, probenecid, sulfinpyrazone, trimethoprim; effects of sulfisoxazole decreased by paraldehyde, para-aminosalicylic acid

10. Anti-inflammatory drugs

   a) Increased effects of insulin, oral anticoagulants and antidiabetics, penicillins, sulfa drugs

   b) Oxyphenbutazone: decreased effects of antihistamines, barbiturates, digitoxin

   c) Prednisone: increased effects of sedatives; decreased effects of coumarin anticoagulants, insulin, oral antidiabetics, pilocarpine; effects of prednisone increased by aspirin, indomethacin; effects of prednisone decreased by antihistamines, chloral hydrate, phenylbutazone, phenytoin, propranolol

11. Antiparkinson drugs

   a) Levodopa: effects decreased by phenothiazines, haloperidol, phenytoin, pyridoxine, reserpine, vitamin B_6 supplements

   b) Amantadine: effects increased by antihistamines, tricyclic antidepressants, phenothiazines

12. Antipsychotics: increased effects of sedatives; decreased effects of levodopa; effects of antipsychotics decreased by antacids, anticholinergics
13. Cardiotonics
    a) Effects of cardiotonics increased by guanethidine, phenytoin, propranolol, quinidine
    b) Effects of cardiotonics decreased by antacids, cholestyramine, kaolin with pectin, laxatives, neomycin, phenobarbital, phenylbutazone, rifampin
    c) Digitalis: risk of toxicity increased by diuretic-induced hypokalemia
14. Diuretics
    a) Increased effects of antihypertensives
    b) Decreased effects of allopurinol, oral antidiabetics and anticoagulants, insulin, probenecid
    c) Effects of diuretics increased by analgesics, barbiturates
    d) Effects of diuretics decreased by aspirin, cholestyramine
15. Laxatives: decreased effects of oral medications
16. Nitrates
    a) Increased effects of atropine, tricyclic antidepressants
    b) Decreased effects of cholinelike drugs
    c) Effects of nitrates increased by alcohol, propranolol
17. Sedatives and hypnotics
    a) Increased effects of analgesics, antihistamines, oral anticoagulants
    b) Decreased effects of corticosteroids
    c) Effects of sedatives and hypnotics decreased by alcohol, antihistamines, phenothiazines

B. Major drug-food interactions
    1. Stimulation or suppression of appetite
       a) Antidepressants, antipsychotics, antianxiety agents, and antihistamines can stimulate appetite.
       b) Anticonvulsants and cardiotonics can suppress appetite.
    2. Alteration in nutrient digestion or absorption
       a) Malabsorption of calcium can occur with ingestion of many antibiotics (e.g., tetracycline).
       b) Some laxatives (e.g., bisacodyl, mineral oil, phenolphthalein) decrease glucose and thiamine uptake.
       c) Mineral oil decreases absorption of vitamins A, D, and K.
       d) Allopurinol decreases iron absorption.
    3. Alteration in metabolism or use of a nutrient
       a) Estrogen increases the breakdown of vitamin C.
       b) Phenytoin increases the breakdown of vitamins D and K.
    4. Alteration in excretion of a nutrient
       a) Thiazide diuretics increase the excretion of calcium, potassium, magnesium, and zinc.
       b) A high-alkaline diet delays the excretion of thioridazine.

I. Pharmacokinetics in the elderly	II. Adverse drug reactions: elderly	III. Drug interactions: elderly	IV. Nursing considerations	V. Alcohol abuse by the elderly

See text pages
_____

IV. Nursing considerations associated with drug use by elderly clients

A. Nursing assessment
  1. Take a complete medication history.
     a) Facilitate history taking by using a 24-hour drug use profile or a review of body systems.
     b) Ask the client to describe the purpose, frequency of administration, and dosage of each drug taken. If possible, have the client bring in all medications so that prescriptions can be checked.
     c) Ask the client to list all over-the-counter (OTC) medications he/she is taking.
     d) Ask about the presence of adverse reactions; factors that may predispose the client to noncompliance; the client's use of caffeine and alcohol; and the client's ability to pay for medications.
  2. Based on the information obtained, further assess problem areas, such as possible adverse effects and drug interactions.

B. Nursing interventions to promote appropriate drug use
  1. Encourage the elderly client to become a more active participant in his/her health care. Have the client ask why a drug has been prescribed, whether it will have any adverse effects, and whether there are any alternatives to drug therapy.
  2. Work with other health care professionals to reduce the number of medications taken by a client and simplify the schedule for taking them.
  3. Make sure that the client receives medication in a container that he/she can open. Inform the client that easy-open containers can be requested at the pharmacy.
  4. Ensure that the client has the visual acuity, educational background, and cognitive ability to read standard medication labels and direction sheets. If not, adapt as needed (e.g., provide large-print materials).
  5. Teach and supervise medication self-administration well before a hospitalized client is to be discharged.
  6. Involve family members or a close friend in teaching sessions whenever possible.
  7. Provide memory aids, such as drug cards, drug calendars, color-coded medication labels and directions, or medication boxes with individual compartments for days of the week and times of day when medication is to be taken.
  8. Be sure the client has the motor skills needed to administer medications (e.g., injections, inhalers, transdermal patches).

V. Alcohol abuse by the elderly

See text pages

A. Problems associated with alcohol abuse
   1. Intellectual deterioration, especially short-term memory and abstract reasoning, particularly when psychoactive drugs are also being taken
   2. Delirium (see Chapter 12, section III,A,1)
   3. Gastrointestinal (GI) problems (e.g., malnutrition, hypoglycemia, lesions, hemorrhage)
   4. Cardiovascular disorders (e.g., enlargement of the heart, arrhythmias, peripheral edema)
   5. Liver disease (increased liver size with reduced function)

B. Nursing considerations associated with alcohol abuse by elderly clients
   1. Nursing assessment
      a) Be alert to the possible presence of alcohol abuse in clients who present with depression, dysplasia, malnutrition, memory impairment, peripheral neuropathy, sleep disorders, or tremors.
      b) Adopt a nonjudgmental manner and ask the client both specific and open-ended questions.
   2. Nursing interventions
      a) Provide supportive care for clients in acute toxic and withdrawal states, stabilizing fluid balance and providing an appropriate level of rest, nutrition, protection, and sedation.
      b) Reassure the client that older people who seek treatment for alcoholism are more likely than younger people to have a successful outcome.
      c) Assist the client in identifying and finding a reimbursement source for an appropriate alcohol treatment program.

1. When a highly fat-soluble drug such as diazepam (Valium) is administered to an elderly client, the nurse should anticipate that:
   a. The dose will need to be increased.
   b. The dose will need to be decreased.
   c. The interval between doses will need to be longer.
   d. The interval between doses will need to be shorter.

2. Mr. Bailey, who has been taking furosemide (Lasix), now has warfarin (Coumadin) prescribed. The nurse will need to be alert for signs of:
   a. Toxicity of both drugs.
   b. Decreased effectiveness of furosemide.
   c. Toxicity of warfarin.
   d. Decreased effectiveness of both drugs.

3. To increase drug effectiveness in the elderly, the nurse should:
   a. Schedule administration of most medications with meals.
   b. Encourage the client to take a full glass of water with each medication.
   c. Schedule administration of most medications at bedtime.
   d. Give medications by injection rather than orally.

4. The risk of adverse reactions to drugs is increased in elderly clients who:
   a. Have recently been hospitalized for an acute illness.
   b. See a physician frequently for management of a chronic illness.
   c. Have been made aware of the potential side effects of medications they take.
   d. Self-treat multiple symptoms with over-the-counter (OTC) medications.

5. Which of the following should alert the nurse that an elderly client is at risk for noncompliance with the prescribed drug regimen?
   a. The client has multiple chronic illnesses.
   b. The client's insurance pays for prescription medications.
   c. The client's prescriptions are renewed by phone and delivered by the pharmacy.
   d. The client stores medications in a cupboard in the kitchen.

6. The client receiving calcium channel-blocking drugs to control blood pressure should be cautioned to anticipate which of the following side effects?
   a. Diarrhea
   b. Drowsiness
   c. Bradycardia
   d. Confusion

7. The risk of aspirin toxicity is increased when aspirin is taken with:
   a. Magaldrate (Riopan).
   b. Propranolol (Inderal).
   c. Penicillin.
   d. Vitamin C.

8. The client who takes oral antidiabetic drugs to control blood sugar should be monitored for hyperglycemia if he/she also receives:
   a. Anticoagulants.
   b. Thiazide diuretics.
   c. Aspirin.
   d. Antidepressants.

9. The client who is receiving both digitalis and a potent diuretic such as furosemide (Lasix) must be closely monitored for:
   a. Digitalis toxicity.
   b. Reduced effectiveness of digitalis.
   c. Kidney damage.
   d. Excessive urine output.

10. The client who takes levodopa (L-Dopa) to control Parkinson's disease should be cautioned to avoid vitamin supplements containing:

   a. Vitamin B$_6$.
   b. Vitamin K.
   c. Vitamin C.
   d. Vitamin D.

11. To assist the elderly person to swallow tablets effectively, the nurse should instruct the client to:

   a. Dissolve the tablet in warm water before taking it.
   b. Crush the tablet and mix it in food.
   c. Place the tablet on the back of the tongue.
   d. Place the tablet on the front of the tongue.

12. It is appropriate to tell the elderly person with an alcohol abuse problem that:

   a. Improved nutrition can alleviate many of the chronic symptoms that develop with alcohol abuse.
   b. Impaired cognition and memory can often be reversed if alcohol use is discontinued.
   c. Elderly clients who seek treatment for alcohol abuse have a higher success rate than younger clients.
   d. Because of the development of tolerance over time, the elderly can often consume large amounts of alcohol before showing symptoms.

ANSWERS

1. Correct answer is c. Because the elderly have increased adipose tissue, the effects of fat-soluble drugs are prolonged. To compensate, doses of the drug should be given further apart.

a and **b.** The need to increase or decrease doses would depend mainly on the individual's body mass. No information to support either choice is given.

d. Since effects of fat-soluble drugs are prolonged, giving doses closer together will increase the risk of toxicity.

2. Correct answer is a. Only a small portion of highly protein-bound drugs such as furosemide or warfarin is expected to be active. When 2 drugs compete for protein-binding sites, more of both is free and active, increasing the toxicity risk.

b and **d.** The effects of both drugs are increased, not decreased; the more active drug is available because the 2 drugs compete for protein-binding sites.
c. It is true that there is greater risk of toxicity of warfarin, but since there is also an increased risk of toxicity of furosemide, **a** is the better answer.

3. Correct answer is b. Adequate fluid intake improves drug absorption and promotes distribution to all body sites. For the client on a fluid-restricted diet, this fluid would have to be planned in the scheduled intake. If the fluid restriction is severe, the amount may have to be reduced.

a. Food delays absorption of most drugs. Medication administration times should generally be 1 hour before or 2 hours after meals.
c. Exercise helps increase absorption of medications. Medications given at bedtime may not be absorbed as well because gastric emptying and circulation to the gastrointestinal (GI) tract are decreased while the client is inactive.
d. Absorption and distribution of injectable forms of drugs are impaired by dehydration and decreased mobility. If these factors are not addressed, use of injectable forms will not increase drug effectiveness.

4. Correct answer is d. The use of multiple OTC medications contributes to polypharmacy in the elderly. Polypharmacy is a major cause of adverse drug reactions.

a. Ongoing treatment of acute or chronic health problems is a risk factor for polypharmacy. A recent hospitalization may have provided the opportunity to review and revise the drug regimen, decreasing adverse interactions.

b. Seeing multiple physicians increases the risk of adverse drug interactions. Frequent visits to 1 physician provide opportunities to evaluate drug effects and may decrease the risk.

c. Clients who know what side effects their medications may cause are less likely to view these side effects as symptoms of a new illness and treat them with other drugs.

5. **Correct answer is c.** When the client's drugs are ordered by phone or mail, the client may fail to receive the necessary instructions to use the medications correctly.

a. Being treated for multiple chronic illnesses increases the risk of polypharmacy with adverse medication effects. It does not necessarily increase the risk of noncompliance.

b. Using insurance to pay for medications may actually increase the likelihood that the client fills all prescriptions. The client who is financially restricted may be unable to fill prescriptions.

d. This may be an appropriate storage place for medications. Having the medications in a room near where the client spends most of his/her time may increase the likelihood of taking them at the prescribed times.

6. **Correct answer is b.** Drowsiness is a common side effect of all antihypertensives, especially in the first few days of use. Tolerance to this effect develops over time.

a. Calcium channel blockers commonly cause constipation.

c. Bradycardia is expected with beta blockers. Calcium channel blockers more often produce tachycardia.

d. Altered cognition is more common with methyldopa or beta blockers. Calcium channel blockers do not commonly alter mental status.

7. **Correct answer is d.** Vitamin C acidifies the urine, decreasing aspirin excretion.

a and **b.** Both magaldrate and propranolol decrease aspirin effects.

c. Aspirin increases the effects of penicillin. The combination is more likely to produce penicillin toxicity than aspirin toxicity.

8. **Correct answer is b.** Thiazide diuretics can decrease the effects of oral antidiabetics, allowing blood sugar to rise.

a and **c.** Both oral anticoagulants and aspirin increase the effects of oral antidiabetics by displacing them from protein-binding sites. The client would most likely become hypoglycemic in this case.

d. No common interaction between antidepressants and antidiabetics is reported.

9. **Correct answer is a.** Hypokalemia induced by diuretics predisposes the client to digitalis toxicity.

b. Diuretics reduce cardiac workload by decreasing blood volume, which is most likely to potentiate digitalis effects.

c. Although some diuretics are nephrotoxic, the combination does not increase this risk. This would not be the most common problem with this combination of drugs.

d. Prolonged use of diuretics can produce dehydration but combining them with digitalis does not increase this risk. Digitalis toxicity is a much more common risk with this combination.

10. **Correct answer is a.** Vitamin B_6 antagonizes the effects of levodopa. No interaction with vitamins C, D, or K is reported.

b. Vitamin K should be avoided by clients taking oral anticoagulants, since it antagonizes their effects.

c. Vitamin C in large doses increases the risk of toxicity with aspirin or acetaminophen.

d. Vitamin D may need to be increased for clients receiving phenytoin, since the drug antagonizes vitamin D's effects.

11. **Correct answer is c.** The surge of fluid swallowed with the tablet is more likely to carry it into the esophagus if the tablet is placed on the back of the tongue.

a and **b.** Dissolving or crushing medications may interfere with drug effectiveness or injure the mucosa that lines the mouth or esophagus. These would not be appropriate first choices.

d. Capsules are appropriately placed on the front of the tongue. This is not appropriate for tablets, which do not float as easily as capsules to the back of the mouth.

12. **Correct answer is c.** Elderly alcoholics have a better prognosis than younger ones. They are more likely to complete treatment and maintain sobriety once they acknowledge the need for treatment.

a. Nutritional deficits contribute to or exacerbate many of the chronic problems produced by alcohol use; these problems, however, may not be reversible with improved nutrition.

b. The mental status changes that result from chronic alcohol use often cannot be reversed, although discontinuing alcohol use can slow their progression.

d. Because of decreased ability to detoxify and excrete alcohol, the elderly are more vulnerable to alcohol's adverse effects.

4

Gerontologic Nursing Settings

NURSING HIGHLIGHTS

1. The nurse should remember that first-time hospitalization may be especially difficult for an older person who may have sensory deficits that impair his/her ability to adapt to new surroundings.
2. The nurse should be aware that the elderly client who is hospitalized may require more attention and assistance than younger clients with tasks such as ambulation, eating, and hygiene.
3. Due to age-related physiologic changes and a reduced margin of physiologic reserve, elderly clients have reduced ability to respond to the stress

of hospitalization and surgery and are at greater risk for surgery-related complications.

4. For many elderly clients, the need to enter a nursing home arises suddenly. The nurse should help clients and their families determine the criteria that are most important to them in selecting a facility.

GLOSSARY

atelectasis—collapse of part or all of the lung

dehiscence—separation of the layers of a surgical wound

evisceration—protrusion of the viscera or internal organs

fistula—an abnormal connection between two internal organs or an internal organ and the surface of the body

Homans' sign—pain at the site of a deep vein thrombosis when the foot is dorsiflexed

keloid—a scar that is elevated, irregularly shaped, and enlarged

nosocomial infection—infection that occurs as a result of exposures during a stay in a health care facility

ENHANCED OUTLINE

I. The elderly client in the acute-care setting

<table>
<tr><td></td><td>See text pages</td></tr>
<tr><td></td><td>_____</td></tr>
</table>

A. General concerns and the role of the nurse
   1. Fear
      a) Issues
         (1) Elderly clients are often apprehensive about being away from home and separated from their spouses and other family members.
         (2) Fear is intensified if the hospitalized person has a family member at home who is in poor health or has trouble caring for himself/herself.
         (3) The hospitalized elderly client may be afraid that he/she will not be able to understand explanations or to follow doctors' and nurses' instructions.
         (4) The elderly client may be apprehensive about being able to care for himself/herself upon discharge from the hospital and may fear placement in a nursing home.
         (5) The elderly client may fear that he/she will be treated in a condescending manner in the hospital.
         (6) The elderly client with mild or moderate cognitive impairments may fear that he/she will be unable to adjust to unfamiliar environments and/or routines.
         (7) Many older people regard hospitals as places to die.

        b) Nursing considerations
           (1) Encourage the client to share his/her feelings about being hospitalized.
           (2) Urge the client to ask questions about the purpose and nature of diagnostic procedures and to ask for clarification if an explanation is not wholly clear.
           (3) Suggest that another family member be present when test results or diagnoses are being discussed.
           (4) Reassure the client about the range of supportive services that will be available postdischarge.
           (5) Encourage the client to verbalize his/her attitude toward hospitals and fears of death.
           (6) Discuss with the client his/her condition while maintaining a positive attitude toward the future.
           (7) Encourage members of the hospital staff to treat the elderly client with courtesy and respect.
    2. Financial concerns
        a) Issues
           (1) Elderly clients, who may already be dealing with financial burdens related to chronic illness, are often concerned about being able to pay for hospital charges not covered by Medicare or private insurance.
           (2) Clients may worry about the cost of transportation, meals, or hotel accommodations for spouses or other family members.
           (3) Elderly clients, particularly those who live on fixed incomes from pensions or Social Security, may be anxious about their ability to pay for postdischarge care.
        b) Nursing considerations
           (1) Refer the client and family to social services or other appropriate source for detailed information about sources of reimbursement available for hospitalization, convalescent facilities, and in-home services.
           (2) Help the client and family identify reasonably priced transportation services, restaurants, and hotels in the vicinity of the hospital.
    3. Confusion and disorientation
        a) Issues
           (1) Factors that cause or enhance confusion for the elderly client may be his/her illness, his/her relocation, changes in sensory input, immobility, pain, polypharmacy, or fear.
           (2) Physical relocation is especially difficult for the client with sensory impairment.

          (3) The elderly client is at high risk for falls, especially early in hospitalization.

   b) Nursing considerations

          (1) Assign the client to a room that is appropriate to his/her physical and mental status (e.g., near the nursing station or, conversely, in a quieter environment).

          (2) Enhance the client's orientation by making sure that he/she knows how to summon a nurse and has a clock and calendar, access to radio and television and, if space permits, family photographs.

          (3) Ascertain the routines the client followed at home (e.g., hour of waking, mealtimes) and try to replicate some of them in the hospital.

          (4) Reassure the elderly client's family that some confusion may be a temporary response to hospitalization and not an indication of dementia onset.

4. Polypharmacy

   a) Issues

          (1) Many elderly clients see multiple physicians who prescribe medications for several conditions.

          (2) Many adverse drug reactions and interactions result from polypharmacy (see sections II,B and III,A of Chapter 3).

          (3) Polypharmacy can exacerbate the disorientation and confusion that many elderly clients experience when they are admitted to the hospital.

   b) Nursing considerations

          (1) Establish the client's drug history.

          (2) Evaluate the client's drug regimen.

          (3) Assess the client's problems as a result of adverse drug reactions or drug interactions.

          (4) Be aware of the client's medication and watch for subtle changes in physical or mental status that may be related to polypharmacy.

5. The client's family

   a) Issues

          (1) Family members, especially the primary caregiver, may be overwhelmed by the seriousness of the client's condition, the financial impact of the illness, and its implications for the future.

          (2) Family members may regard the client's hospitalization as an indication that they did not devote enough time or attention to the hospitalized individual.

          (3) Family members may feel displaced in the presence of highly trained health care professionals.

   b) Nursing considerations

          (1) Be attentive to the needs of the client's family, especially those of the primary caregiver.

             (2) Keep family members informed of the client's progress; if necessary, arrange for other members of the health care team to meet with the family and answer their questions.

             (3) Help family members to keep the client's illness in perspective; when appropriate, refer them to social services or to a hospital chaplain.

             (4) Include the family in the client's care plan and encourage them to help the client remain as independent as possible.

B. Hospital-related medical problems
1. Pressure sores and other integumentary disorders
   a) Predisposing factors
      (1) Immobility or reduced mobility
      (2) Subclinical malnutrition
      (3) Anemia
      (4) Reduced peripheral circulation
      (5) Skin infections, dry skin, and pruritus and the loss of skin elasticity
   b) Nursing considerations
      (1) Assess serum albumin level upon admission (<2.6 g may indicate risk for pressure sores).
      (2) See that the client at high risk for pressure sores has a diet high in carbohydrates, proteins, and vitamins and increased fluid intake.
      (3) Assist the client in ambulating for short distances, sitting in a chair, and changing positions at least every 2 hours.
      (4) Reposition the client by lifting rather than dragging or sliding, and gently massage bony areas.
      (5) If available, use pressure-relieving devices (e.g., alternating-pressure or air mattresses, air-fluidized devices).
      (6) Monitor the incontinent client for wetness and gently cleanse skin exposed to urine or feces with warm water and mild soap.
      (7) Immediately report any reddened area of the skin that does not return to normal skin color after pressure is relieved; it may be an early sign of pressure sores.
      (8) Do not massage preulcer areas, but relieve pressure as much as possible. Use protective padding for bony prominences.
      (9) Encourage the hospitalized client with dry skin or pruritus to rehydrate the dermis with bath oils or emollients and to avoid scratching.

2. Nosocomial infections: most commonly affect the respiratory, gastrointestinal, genitourinary, and integumentary systems
   a) Predisposing factors
      (1) Immobility
      (2) Tissue damage
      (3) Use of a Foley catheter, intravenous (IV) cannula, or other invasive device
      (4) Use of drugs that suppress the immune system
      (5) Circulatory impairment (e.g., peripheral vascular disease)
      (6) Diabetes mellitus
      (7) Anemia
   b) Nursing considerations
      (1) Follow infection control procedures carefully.
      (2) Be especially alert to early signs of infection, because usual signs (e.g., elevated temperature) are often depressed, late, or absent in elderly clients.
      (3) Recognize that mental status changes are often the first sign of infection in the elderly.
3. Falls: occur most frequently at night or while the client is getting in or out of bed or being transferred to a wheelchair
   a) Predisposing factors
      (1) Osteoporosis or other bone-weakening condition
      (2) Musculoskeletal disorders that require use of ambulatory assistance devices
      (3) Poor balance
      (4) Orthostatic hypotension
      (5) Disorientation, confusion, or cognitive impairment
      (6) Nocturia
      (7) Use of physical restraints or full bedside rails
      (8) Administration of sedatives, laxatives, diuretics, and antihypertensive agents
      (9) Incontinence
   b) Nursing considerations
      (1) Orient the client to place at least once each shift during the first 3 days of hospitalization or as needed.
      (2) Provide frequent reminders of how to call for assistance.
      (3) At night, keep a night light or the bathroom light on in the client's room.
      (4) Ensure that all staff use proper transfer techniques from bed and wheelchair.
      (5) Help the client get regular physical exercise; if he/she cannot ambulate, assist with passive or active range-of-motion exercises.
      (6) Use a raised chair seat and other adapted furniture that are at the right height for the client.
      (7) Use side rails only for the top half of the client's bed and use physical restraints only as a last resort.

    4. Incontinence: urinary and fecal
        a) Predisposing factors (see also Chapter 1, sections VIII,A,1 and VIII,A,2,c)
           (1) Confusion, disorientation, emotional upset, or dementia
           (2) Severe illness
           (3) Inconvenient location of the toilet or fear of going to the toilet
           (4) Difficulty in manipulating clothing or using a urinal or bedpan
        b) Nursing considerations
           (1) Ensure that the client knows how to summon the nurse.
           (2) Ensure that the client has access to a toilet or to an appropriate toilet substitute (commode, overtoilet chair, bedpan, or urinal).
           (3) Administer drugs as prescribed for urinary incontinence (e.g., flavoxate, oxybutynin, pseudoephedrine).
           (4) Use Foley and condom catheters only as a last resort for urinary incontinence.
           (5) Unless contraindicated, encourage the client with fecal incontinence to drink 2 liters of fluid per day and to consume 6–10 g of fiber.
           (6) Help the client identify triggers that cause fecal incontinence.
           (7) Assist the client to the bathroom and provide privacy at the client's usual time for fecal elimination.
           (8) As a last resort, provide protective undergarments for the client with fecal incontinence.

  C. Preoperative care of the elderly client (see Client Teaching Checklist, "Preadmission Behaviors That Can Reduce the Risk of Postsurgical Complications in the Elderly Client")
    1. General nursing assessment
        a) Gather baseline data on all body systems.
        b) Note especially the condition of the client's extremities, skin and teeth, range of motion, and affect.
        c) Ascertain the client's current ability to perform activities of daily living (ADLs), the appropriateness and safety of the home environment, and the family's ability and willingness to provide postsurgical care.
    2. Maintenance of adequate hydration and nutrition
        a) Assess the client for signs of subclinical malnutrition or dehydration.
        b) Record recent weight loss and hematocrit and hemoglobin values.

Preadmission Behaviors That Can Reduce the Risk of Postsurgical Complications in the Elderly Client

To reduce the high risk for surgical complications, make the following suggestions to the client when initial arrangements for elective surgery are being made.

✔ Drink at least 2 liters of fluid every day to prevent constipation.
✔ Eat a well-balanced diet.
✔ Take dietary supplements as directed; do not increase the dosage on your own.
✔ To decrease the risk of respiratory complications, stop smoking or drastically reduce the number of cigarettes you smoke during the week before surgery.
✔ Maintain your normal level of physical activity during the days before surgery.
✔ Make a list of any drugs that you take during the week before surgery—prescription drugs, over-the-counter medications, vitamin and mineral supplements, and home remedies and tonics—and bring it with you to the hospital.

  c) Encourage a well-balanced high-protein diet (unless contraindicated by the client's condition).
  d) Measure fluid intake and output.
  e) If necessary, replace fluids and electrolytes by intravenous (IV) administration.
3. Management of physical disorders
  a) Document the presence of health problems that are unrelated to the reason for surgery (e.g., arthritis, benign prostatic hypertrophy, cataracts, chronic obstructive pulmonary disease, circulatory problems, diabetes, hypertension, osteoporosis, presbycusis, urinary tract infections).
  b) Determine the ways in which these conditions will affect the client's perioperative nursing care. Be aware that underlying pulmonary disease, reduced cardiovascular function, and renal disease put the elderly person at high risk for postoperative complications.
4. Management and modification of the medication regimen
  a) Ascertain whether the client has been taking any drugs that have not already been reported to the physician.
  b) Take special note of medications that may cause complications during the perioperative period (e.g., anticoagulants, anticholinergic agents, antidepressants, aspirin, bromides, corticosteroids, nonsteroidal anti-inflammatory drugs [NSAIDs]). Be aware that nephrotoxic antibiotics and alpha-adrenergic vasopressor agents may lead to postoperative renal failure.
  c) Review with the physician those medications the client is receiving that should be continued throughout the perioperative period.

     5. Physical preparation
       a) Perform standard preoperative procedures, taking special care to reduce risk of infection.
         (1) Do not damage the client's skin during shaving.
         (2) Do not apply lubricants to the skin, which will encourage the retention of bacteria.
         (3) Encourage good oral hygiene in case of perioperative trauma to the oral cavity.
       b) Observe for and report loose teeth to the physician.
       c) Apply elastic stockings to prevent postoperative embolism as ordered.
       d) Pad bony prominences.
       e) If an enema or laxatives are ordered, assist with toileting as needed to prevent falls.
       f) The night before surgery, administer a short-acting sedative or hypnotic as ordered. Elderly clients may need ⅓–½ the adult dose because of increased sensitivity to these drugs.
       g) Remain with the client after administration of a sedative or hypnotic to monitor for temporary confusion or disorientation.
     6. Psychologic preparation
       a) Reduce anxiety in the client and the family.
         (1) Describe the surgical experience the client can expect.
         (2) Discuss the severity and type of expected postsurgical pain and means of managing it.
         (3) Have the client practice techniques for minimizing postsurgical complications (turning, deep breathing, and coughing).
         (4) Demonstrate expected postsurgical procedures (e.g., oxygen administration, catheter use, suctioning, dressing changes).
       b) Encourage the client and family to ask questions and allow adequate time to discuss their concerns.
       c) Arrange for a visit by a hospital chaplain, if appropriate.

   D. Intraoperative care of the elderly client
     1. Prevention of hypothermia
       a) Be aware that older clients are at high risk for perioperative hypothermia because of decreases in metabolic rate and the effects of anesthesia.
       b) Keep the client adequately covered in the holding area and operating room.
     2. Appropriate movement and positioning
       a) Position the client on the operating table slowly and carefully, remembering that osteoporosis and limited range of motion may be present.

b) Make sure that the extremities are not cramped or resting in a poor position or against equipment or wrinkled bedding.
3. Skin cleaning and preparation
    a) Clean and prep the skin carefully, using a solution that causes minimal irritation.
    b) Use paper tape, as it causes less skin damage than other types, and provide counter traction while removing tape.
    c) Note if a particular position has been maintained for a long period of time so that affected areas can be monitored for the development of pressure sores.
4. Concerns associated with anesthesia
    a) Due to age-related changes, less anesthetic is required to produce anesthesia in elderly clients than in younger adults, and the elderly require more time to eliminate anesthetics.
    b) Verbal assurances should be provided if the client has received regional, local, or spinal anesthesia and is awake. Local anesthesia is better tolerated by the elderly client than general anesthesia.

E. Postoperative care of the elderly client
    1. Care of the respiratory system
        a) Maintain a patent airway by proper positioning of the client, preventing aspiration, and keeping airways free of secretions.
        b) Prevent hypoxia by avoiding a supine position and administering oxygen, if necessary; changes in mental status (e.g., restlessness, delirium) are possible signs of hypoxia. Restlessness must not be taken for a sign of pain as narcotics will deplete oxygen in the body.
        c) Prevent atelectasis and hypostatic pneumonia by positioning the client so that the rib cage can expand easily and the diaphragm can descend.
        d) Adopt a regimen designed to prevent respiratory complications and excessive central nervous system depression as soon as the client's vital signs begin to stabilize; e.g., turn the client every 2 hours and encourage deep breathing and coughing.
        e) Use chest physical therapy, postural drainage, incentive spirometry, and intermittent positive pressure breathing if required.
    2. Care of the cardiovascular and peripheral vascular systems
        a) Take vital signs frequently; abnormal values may signal the development of postsurgical complications (e.g., shock, hemorrhage).
        b) Assess for signs of thrombophlebitis (see Nurse Alert, "Measures for Preventing Thrombophlebitis").
        c) Be particularly alert to warning signals of myocardial infarction (e.g., vague, nonspecific pain).
        d) Monitor fluid administration carefully; elderly clients may develop congestive heart failure secondary to normal postoperative fluid shifts.

3. Care of the renal system
   a) Maintain strict records of fluid intake and output, and assess them regularly for acute renal failure and signs of oliguria and anuria.
   b) Due to the risk of infection, do not catheterize the client unless necessary; palpate and percuss for bladder distention to determine the need for catheterization.
   c) To facilitate voiding, ensure the client's privacy; help men stand up, and assist women to sitting position on bedpan or commode.
   d) Monitor the client for signs of electrolyte and acid-base imbalances, which may lead to arrhythmias.
4. Management of postoperative confusion
   a) Be especially alert to the development of postoperative confusion or delirium in clients with characteristics associated with increased susceptibility (e.g., signs of impaired cognition on admission, extreme old age, decreased postoperative mobility, urinary problems).
   b) Rule out hypoxia, infections, and fluid, electrolyte, and acid-base imbalances as soon as signs of confusion are noted.
   c) Encourage reorientation by calling the client by name, allowing the client to wear eyeglasses or a hearing aid unless

! NURSE *ALERT* !

Measures for Preventing Thrombophlebitis

Thrombophlebitis is a common surgical complication in elderly clients and can progress to pulmonary embolism, the most frequent cause of postoperative death among the elderly. To reduce the risk of thrombophlebitis, take the following measures.

- Apply antiembolism stockings, and remove them for 1 hour each shift.
- Ensure that the client exercises the ankles and legs every hour. Use passive range-of-motion exercises if the client cannot perform active exercises.
- Help the client ambulate as soon as possible.
- Avoid applying any kind of pressure under the client's knees, such as that caused by crossing the legs or placing a pillow under the knees.
- Frequently monitor the color, temperature, circulation, sensation, and movement of each leg.
- Check both calves at regular intervals for signs of thrombophlebitis (e.g., redness, heat, pain, positive Homans' sign, swelling). Measuring the calves is an effective way to confirm the presence of swelling.

contraindicated, explaining the care that is being given, and encouraging the client to make as many decisions as possible.

5. Management of postoperative pain
   a) Administer analgesics immediately as needed.
   b) Use medications that do not have long half-lives or active metabolites because the elderly do not tolerate pain medication well due to slower metabolism.
   c) Administration of small doses at regular intervals may help reduce the incidence of adverse effects of higher doses (e.g., suppression of cough reflex), but the elderly client needs to receive enough analgesic to perform deep breathing and coughing without pain.
   d) Encourage the client to request an analgesic when he/she perceives pain.
   e) Use nonnarcotic analgesics (e.g., acetaminophen) in conjunction with narcotics.
   f) Administer a narcotic antagonist (e.g., naloxone hydrochloride) if the client exhibits signs of respiratory depression.
   g) Supplement the administration of analgesics with comfort-promoting measures (e.g., back rubs, hot tea, relaxation techniques, guided imagery).

6. Maintaining body temperature
   a) To reduce the high risk for hypothermia among the elderly, ensure that the client's environment is sufficiently warm and that he/she is adequately covered.
   b) Use rewarming devices (e.g., hypothermia blanket, warming mattress, radiant heat lamps) to return body temperature to normal in the recovery room.

7. Facilitating wound healing: Be aware that wound healing usually occurs more slowly in elderly clients.
   a) Watch for the presence of abnormal laboratory values (e.g., low serum albumin, elevated blood glucose) that are often associated with wound-healing complications.
   b) Learn to recognize early signs of common complications of wound healing (e.g., formation of fistulas or keloids, scarring, wound herniation, dehiscence, evisceration).
   c) Check often for an increase in serous drainage or nonapproximation of wound edges; these may be signs of dehiscence and evisceration, which are emergency situations.

8. Care of the gastrointestinal system: Be aware that paralytic ileus is often prolonged in elderly clients as is their progress from clear liquids to solids.
   a) Maintain fluid and electrolyte balance intravenously until bowel sounds are detected.
   b) Prevent gastrointestinal problems by offering small, frequent feedings rather than 3 substantial meals.
   c) Encourage the client to eat his/her favorite foods unless contraindicated by his/her condition.

          d) Treat postsurgical constipation by increasing the client's consumption of fluids and dietary fiber.

          e) Assist with early ambulation to speed return of peristalsis.

  F. Care of the elderly client in the intensive care unit (ICU)

    1. Psychosocial needs: Prompt attention to the psychosocial needs of the critically ill older adult may minimize or prevent depression, passivity, disorientation, confusion, fear, frustration, or hostility that may stem from feeling helpless or hopeless.

      a) Encourage the critically ill client who is able to participate to share questions and concerns.

      b) Discourage family members from speaking for the client unless he/she cannot speak.

      c) Reassure critically ill older adults that everything will be done to restore their previous level of health and to help them regain their independence.

      d) Attempt to confirm all nonverbal cues (e.g., facial grimaces) with the client rather than assuming their meaning.

      e) Try to determine the basis for the client's emotional state and help him/her to view the situation from a realistic but hopeful perspective.

      f) Respect the clients and protect their privacy by ensuring that they are well screened before their bodies are exposed and that inappropriate conversations do not take place in their presence, even if they appear to be asleep or unconscious.

    2. Response to disease

      a) Observe the critically ill client for subtle signs of infection: temperature >98.6°F, a pronounced change in mental status, a change in an underlying condition (e.g., diabetes mellitus), symptoms of dehydration, or elevated white blood cell (WBC) count or blood urea nitrogen (BUN) levels.

      b) Be especially vigilant for the presence of superinfection on the fourth or fifth day of antibiotic therapy. Assess for bloody diarrhea and/or white patches in the mouth.

      c) Guard against hypothermia in the critically ill older person by keeping the ambient temperature of the ICU warm, keeping the client appropriately dressed and well covered, and having a cap available to protect against heat loss from the head.

    3. Fluid balance and nutrition

      a) Maintain fluid balance.

        (1) Offer fluids at frequent intervals, and encourage the family to do so as well.

        (2) Monitor intake and output.

      b) Maintain adequate nutrition.
         (1) Weigh the client at appropriate intervals; do it before breakfast.
         (2) Keep accurate calorie counts, if appropriate.
         (3) Enhance the pleasure of meals by encouraging family members to be present.
         (4) Schedule the administration of analgesics so that the client is pain-free at mealtimes.
  4. Cardiac and respiratory risks
      a) Monitor the critically ill older client for atypical signs of heart failure (e.g., weakness, apprehension, confusion, somnolence).
      b) Control intravenous (IV) therapy carefully, because the heart of the critically ill older adult may have limited ability to compensate for rapid fluid shifts.
      c) Encourage the client to ambulate as soon as possible to prevent the deconditioning of the heart and muscles that occurs with bed rest. Assist with active range-of-motion exercises if the client cannot ambulate.
      d) In the client who is receiving antihypertensive medication, monitor for orthostatic hypotension, a major risk factor for falls.
      e) Maintain pulmonary hygiene in the critically ill client by encouraging coughing, deep breathing, turning, and early ambulation.
      f) Encourage the client to sit up while eating or receiving tube feedings to lessen the risk of aspiration.
G. Discharge planning
  1. Assessing the client's learning abilities
      a) Recognize that the elderly client's ability to learn may be impaired by distractions (e.g., noise).
      b) Determine the presence of age-related physical changes that may affect the client's ability to learn self-care measures (e.g., hearing and vision impairments, inability to read) or that may affect the client's attention span (e.g., impaired thermoregulation, persistent pain).
      c) Assess for the presence of sensory deficits that may impair the performance of self-care activities; e.g., an impaired sense of smell would indicate to the nurse that teaching the client to recognize the presence of a urinary tract infection by a change in the smell of urine would not be effective.
      d) Determine the presence of viewpoints that may compromise the client's willingness to learn or make lifestyle modifications.
         (1) The conviction that daily life is too difficult and complex to allow for the addition of a new routine
         (2) The client's impression that he/she does not have the educational background to learn to manage a chronic disease like diabetes

I. The elderly client in the acute-care setting	II. The elderly client at home	III. The elderly client in a nursing facility

         (3) The belief that fate is in control and cannot be affected by self-care activities

    e) Determine how much the client already knows about his/her medical problem and whether he/she has misconceptions about the condition or its treatment.

    f) Ask the elderly client whether he/she prefers reading material, listening to presentations or audiotapes, or participating in "hands-on" workshops.

    g) Determine the client's level of literacy by using listening tests and word recognition tests.

2. Enhancing learning in elderly clients

    a) Allow adequate time to define teaching priorities and learning goals with the client, to select or prepare instructional materials, to conduct teaching session(s), to evaluate the client's learning, to correct areas of misunderstanding, to revise teaching strategies, and to conduct follow-up teaching session(s).

    b) Tailor the pace of presentations and the length of learning sessions to the capabilities and health status of the client.

    c) Foster the client's belief that he/she is capable of self-care by recognizing each effort and achievement, avoiding any behavior that would threaten the client's self-esteem, and providing liberal praise.

    d) Facilitate learning by breaking down each skill (e.g., self-administration of insulin) into manageable subtasks.

    e) Establish a mentor-protégé relationship with the client to create the atmosphere of mutual trust conducive to learning.

    f) Conduct learning sessions in a well-lit, glare-free, quiet, and comfortable environment.

    g) Make use of techniques that enhance memory (e.g., imaging techniques, mnemonics, repetition, sensory stimulation, restatement and rewriting, analogies). Provide the client with written memory aids that he/she can keep.

    h) If the client is receptive, use newer teaching devices (e.g., videotapes, audiotapes, computers) to enhance learning.

    i) Make alternate arrangements if the nursing schedule does not allow sufficient time for teaching of the hospitalized client.

3. Ensuring continuity of care

    a) Offer a variety of resources that clients and families can choose from to ensure that their needs are met appropriately.

    b) Enlist input from other members of the health care team when developing a discharge plan: client, family, physicians, nurses, pharmacists, social workers, nutritionists, therapists (occupational, physical, and speech), and chaplains.

c) Prepare a plan that addresses the following issues:
   (1) Where the client will go when he/she leaves the hospital
   (2) The client's ability to manage activities of daily living (ADLs) and instrumental activities of daily living (IADLs)
   (3) The client's physical and mental status
   (4) Medications and treatments that will be required
   (5) The client's existing support system
   (6) The client's current health and social service needs
   (7) People or agencies that will meet the client's needs
   (8) Success of the teaching that has been done with the client and/or family as well as additional teaching needs
   (9) Equipment and supplies that are needed
   (10) Appropriate referrals for the client and the financial implications of such referrals
   (11) Choices that were presented to the client and family; preferences expressed by them
   (12) People who made and received referrals
   (13) Person responsible for coordinating follow-up care
4. Principles of case management
   a) Case management involves coordinating needed services as a follow-up to discharge planning.
   b) Case management provides home- and community-based services that allow the older adult to remain independent in the community.
   c) The most important goals of case management are prevention of premature institutionalization, improved continuity of care, enhanced quality of life for the caregiver, elimination of barriers to obtaining health care services, and reduction of expenditures for long-term care.

II. The elderly client at home

A. Adapting the home environment for the elderly client
   1. Assess the client's home for conditions that might increase the risk of fire hazards.
      a) Make specific recommendations for eliminating hazards.
      b) Make sure that the home has a smoke detector and hand-held fire extinguisher.
      c) Establish a schedule for changing smoke detector batteries.
   2. Determine environmental adaptations that should be made to enhance client mobility and reduce the risk of falls (e.g., installing an outdoor ramp; increasing access to kitchen counters and to the toilet, bathtub, and bathroom sink; widening doorways so that wheelchairs can pass through; raising the height of the bed; anchoring area rugs; marking the edges of steps and other changes in floor height).
   3. Assess the client's needs for special equipment and supplies that will help maintain the client at home (e.g., bathroom grab bars,

See text pages
_____

respiratory devices, rehabilitation equipment, hospital beds, hydraulic lifts, home dialysis equipment).
4. Consider the installation of an emergency response system for the frail older person who lives alone.
5. Provide information about grants and loans that are available for major renovations.

B. Supportive services for clients with moderately impaired self-care capacity
   1. Chore services: light housekeeping, minor repair, errand, and shopping services available through local social service departments, health departments, private homemaker agencies, and religious organizations
   2. Meal services: meal delivery services available through departments of social services, health departments, offices on aging, and religious organizations
   3. Telephone reassurance programs: daily telephone contact to ensure that the client is safe and to provide regular social interaction, conducted by local health or social service agencies or the local chapter of the American Red Cross

C. Partial and intermittent care services for clients with seriously impaired self-care capacity
   1. Day treatment centers (also called adult day care centers)
      a) Programs with recreational, nutritional, and health components designed for clients with serious physical or cognitive impairments
      b) Also intended to afford respite for caregivers
   2. Home care services
      a) Foster care and group home services: services to individuals who retain some self-care capacity but require continuous supervision
      b) Sheltered housing: apartment complexes that supplement independent living in accessible, hazard-free units, with communal meals, health programs, and monitoring services
   3. Hospice programs: a program of support and palliative care for terminally ill clients and their families that may be based in the client's home or situated within a larger institution

See text pages

_____

III. The elderly client in a nursing facility

A. Identifying elderly clients who need a nursing facility
   1. Clients over age 65 who have 2 or more chronic conditions causing functional disability (e.g., limited mobility and incontinence, accompanied by psychologic changes)

2. Clients who need specialized care on a long-term basis (e.g., those with tracheostomies, gastrostomies, and cystostomies; those who require prolonged IV therapy)
3. Clients with a history of coronary thrombosis, cerebrovascular accidents, arthritis, osteoporosis, diabetes, blindness, and emphysema
4. Clients with a history of organic mental disorders, severe confusion, depression, and dementia
5. Clients who are recovering from major surgical procedures (e.g., surgery for malignancies, hip or knee replacements)

B. Types of nursing facilities
1. May be freestanding, a section of a life-care retirement center, or a unit in a state mental hospital (for clients with serious psychiatric or cognitive impairments)
2. May be owned by a corporation, religious group, fraternal organization, or union
3. May have either for-profit or nonprofit status
4. May be government-approved to receive Medicaid and/or Medicare funds

C. Considerations in selecting a facility
1. Philosophy of care: stresses rehabilitation and restorative measures rather than custodial care; has a policy about care of the terminally ill that is consistent with the client's wishes (e.g., a policy that advance directives will be respected)
2. Treatment of clients: promotes client safety, hygiene, and independence; encourages clients and their families to participate in their care
3. Condition of the physical plant: is safe, clean, and attractive; has bright, cheerful rooms and dining area
4. Level of care: has the expertise to care for clients with special medical needs (e.g., use of ventilators); provides adjunct services to enhance the client's health and comfort (e.g., podiatry services, physical therapy, speech therapy); has a low incidence of medical complications (e.g., pressure ulcers, dehydration, falls); can meet the dietary needs of the client and serves high-quality, high-variety meals; offers frequent, varied activities
5. Staffing issues: has an adequate number of caregivers on all shifts; has an average or below-average rate of staff turnover; has high-quality client-staff interactions; has well-qualified staff physicians; has consultant pharmacists; has an appropriate ratio of registered nurses, licensed practical nurses, and nursing assistants; offers the client's family access to the administrator, medical director, director of nursing, and department heads
6. Personal considerations: is close to family members and friends so they can visit the client frequently, is in a safe location, has the resources to meet the client's religious or spiritual needs

7. Financial considerations: per diem rate and the cost of other services that the client will require, types of health insurance that are accepted, the continuing out-of-pocket costs that will be needed to supplement insurance, the status of the client if reimbursement limits are reached, ownership and financial soundness

D. Common nursing care concerns in the long-term-care facility
 1. The nurse must be continuously vigilant for any type of disrespectful or abusive behavior toward a client, intervene immediately to stop it, and report it to the appropriate person.
 2. Because most nursing-home care is given by unlicensed personnel, nurses must monitor the competence of staff, correct performance problems, and devote significant time to staff education.
 3. Since the nursing home is not continuously staffed by physicians and pharmacists, the nurse has responsibility for assessing and monitoring client problems and must act as resident client advocate.
 4. The nurse must be alert to the medical emergencies that commonly occur in nursing homes (e.g., myocardial infarction, cardiac arrest, cerebrovascular accident, acute closed-angle glaucoma, respiratory and urinary tract infections, choking, falls).
 5. Because many nursing home residents will die in the facility, the nurse must explore his/her own feelings about death and dying in order to be able to give the highest level of support to the dying client and the client's family.

1. The elderly client's adjustment to hospitalization is promoted by:
   a. Allowing the client to keep routine medications at the bedside.
   b. Reassuring the client that there is no need to worry about hospital fees before discharge.
   c. Storing the client's belongings in drawers or closets to prevent clutter.
   d. Encouraging the client's family to assist with some of the client's care.

2. To reduce the risk of pressure sores in the hospitalized elderly client, the nurse should:
   a. Massage reddened areas at each position change.
   b. Assist the client to change position every 4 hours.
   c. Use a draw sheet to reposition the client.
   d. Substitute high-protein snacks for those high in carbohydrates.

3. When an elderly client with diabetes has invasive treatments using intravenous (IV) infusions or Foley catheters, it is especially important that the nurse monitor him/her for which of the following early signs of infection?
   a. Elevated temperature
   b. Altered mental status
   c. Purulent drainage
   d. Fluid volume deficit

4. Which of the following nursing actions will help most to reduce the hospitalized elderly client's risk of falling?
   a. Make sure full side rails are used at all times.
   b. Restrain the client with a jacket restraint at night.
   c. Assist the client to get regular exercise.
   d. Keep the call signal where the client can reach it.

5. To reduce the risk of surgical complications, the nurse should instruct the elderly client to do which of the following during the week prior to elective surgery?
   a. Limit fluid intake to 1500 cc daily.
   b. Take supplemental iron and vitamin C.
   c. Avoid vigorous exercise and increase rest periods.
   d. Consume adequate dietary protein and fiber.

6. Appropriate preoperative care for the elderly client includes:
   a. Moisturizing the skin with lubricating lotion.
   b. Avoiding the use of mouthwash.
   c. Encouraging the client to practice techniques for turning and coughing.
   d. Avoiding administration of sedatives within 24 hours of surgery.

7. To prevent postoperative thromboembolism, the nurse should assist the elderly client to:
   a. Apply antiembolism stockings before getting out of bed.
   b. Exercise the legs and ankles hourly.
   c. Support the knees in a flexed position with pillows.
   d. Maintain the legs in a fully extended position.

8. Which of the following should alert the nurse to the presence of wound dehiscence in the elderly client?
   a. An increase in serous drainage
   b. Redness at the wound edges
   c. Itching around the wound
   d. Yellow or green drainage around the sutures

9. To detect superinfection in critically ill elderly clients who have been receiving antibiotics, the nurse should assess for:

    a. Purulent vaginal drainage.
    b. White patches in the mouth.
    c. Mild temperature elevation.
    d. Foul odor to the urine.

10. Discharge teaching for an elderly client is most likely to be effective if:

    a. Multiple teaching sessions are planned.
    b. Teaching is deferred until recovery is complete.
    c. Teaching methods make use of the client's strongest sensory function.
    d. Teaching is done in a group setting.

11. One of the most important goals of case management is to:

    a. Avoid hospital stays.
    b. Reduce insurance costs to the public.
    c. Establish standards for long-term care.
    d. Increase continuity of care.

12. For which client would admission to a nursing facility be most essential?

    a. A client with more than 1 chronic illness
    b. A client who is recovering after a total hip replacement
    c. A client whose cardiac status prevents the performance of housework
    d. A terminally ill client

ANSWERS

1. **Correct answer is d.** Research demonstrates increased satisfaction with care when the family is permitted to participate. The client may accept care from a familiar provider more easily than from hospital staff.

    a. Any medications the client takes may interact with new medications prescribed in the hospital. Scheduling or dosage of these medications may need to be adjusted to assure compatibility. It is important that nurses be aware of all medications taken by the client and their timing.
    b. Worry about financial considerations may impede the client's recovery. It is important to help the client obtain accurate information about fees and payment methods as soon as such concerns are raised.
    c. Having familiar belongings where they are visible will promote adjustment to the new environment. Such belongings should not be stored out of the client's reach.

2. **Correct answer is c.** A draw sheet should be used to avoid sliding or dragging the elderly client, which would cause damaging friction to skin surfaces.

    a. Reddened areas that do not disappear after pressure is relieved are the first sign of pressure ulcers. Massage could further damage the underlying tissues and should be avoided.
    b. Position changes should be made every 2 hours.
    d. It is important to increase dietary protein, but this should not be done at the expense of carbohydrates. Carbohydrates are necessary to spare protein for tissue repair.

3. **Correct answer is b.** Mental status changes are often the first sign of infection in the elderly.

    a and c. The usual signs of infection, such as fever or purulent drainage, are often depressed, late, or absent in the elderly. The nurse must be alert for less common signs that appear earlier.
    d. Fluid volume deficit is not an early sign of infection. It would develop following a period of fever or poor intake.

4. **Correct answer is c.** Regular exercise, which promotes adequate circulation and maintains muscle strength, will decrease the likelihood of falls due to weakness or hypotension.

    a. Half rails are a better choice for the elderly, who may attempt to climb over rails when they need to get up.

b. Restraints are a last resort, since they may add to confusion and agitation, thus increasing the risk of falls.

d. Merely placing the signal within reach does not assure that the client will understand how to use it. The hospitalized elderly client needs to be reminded frequently of how and when to use the signal.

5. **Correct answer is d.** A well-balanced diet, with appropriate levels of protein and fiber, is important to promote wound healing and prevent complications. The client would, of course, be NPO on the night prior to surgery.

a. It is important to maintain a fluid intake of 2000 cc or more to reduce the risk of constipation or dehydration.

b. Dietary supplements should be used only as prescribed by the physician. Since iron supplements cause constipation, they should be avoided unless they are actually needed.

c. The client should maintain normal levels of exercise to promote adequate respiratory and circulatory function.

6. **Correct answer is c.** The client should practice any techniques that will be used postoperatively to assure familiarity with them when they are required.

a. Application of lubricants to the skin should be avoided preoperatively because they promote bacterial growth on the skin.

b. Good mouth care is necessary in case of damage to the mucosa in the intraoperative period. Mouthwash may reduce the number of microorganisms in the oral cavity, which helps prevent infection.

d. Sedatives are often appropriate to manage preoperative anxiety, although doses may need to be reduced for the elderly.

7. **Correct answer is b.** Hourly exercise of the legs and ankles, whether by ambulation or range-of-motion exercises, decreases the risk of thromboembolism.

a. Antiembolism stockings should be worn both in and out of bed to prevent thromboembolism. They should be removed briefly once a shift, but left in place the rest of the time.

c. Nothing should be placed behind the client's knees, since pressure on this area increases the risk of venous stasis and thrombus formation.

d. Full extension of the legs may be uncomfortable and does nothing to reduce the risk of thromboembolism.

8. **Correct answer is a.** Increased serous drainage or nonapproximation of wound edges signals possible wound dehiscence, which requires emergency intervention.

b. Redness of the wound edges appears in the inflammatory phase of wound healing and is not abnormal.

c. Itching around the wound is common during the healing process.

d. Green or yellow drainage is most likely purulent, signaling wound infection.

9. **Correct answer is b.** White patches in the mouth are indicative of thrush, which is a superinfection with *Candida albicans*.

a. White vaginal drainage and itching are signs of vaginal candidiasis, which may be a superinfection. Purulent drainage, however, is more likely to reflect a primary bacterial infection.

c. Fever may be a reaction to the drug or a sign of the underlying infection. It is seldom indicative of superinfection.

d. Foul urine odor would be a sign of urinary tract infection (UTI). UTI is a common nosocomial infection but seldom occurs as a superinfection.

10. **Correct answer is a.** It is important to limit the content covered in a single session to suit the client's attention span and physical endurance. It is best to provide at least 1 follow-up session in which misconceptions can be identified and questions answered.

b. If teaching is delayed until recovery is complete, there may not be adequate time to meet the client's needs. Elderly clients need extra time to learn new material.

c. The elderly client is more likely to learn effectively when all of the senses are stimulated.

d. Group sessions may be too distracting for an elderly client. A quiet environment free of noise and other distractions will facilitate learning for most elderly clients.

11. **Correct answer is d.** Important goals of case management include greater continuity of care, enhanced quality of life for care-givers, prevention of premature institution-alization, and reduction of expenditures for long-term care.

a. Case management goals include preventing premature institutionalization, not avoidance of hospital admissions.

b. Case management aims to reduce expenditures for long-term care, not insurance costs.

c. Establishing standards for long-term care was a function of the Omnibus Budget Reconciliation Act (OBRA), which regulates long-term care. It is not a goal of case management.

12. **Correct answer is b.** Clients recovering from major surgeries require the intensive rehabilitative services that a nursing facility can provide. Such an intense rehabilitation schedule would be difficult, if not impossible, to maintain at home.

a. Chronic illnesses do not necessitate care in a nursing facility unless they are accompanied by functional disabilities.

c. This client would benefit from supportive homemaker services at home since the client has the ability to perform basic activities of daily living (ADLs).

d. Hospice services, which provide symptom management and support services, are available to permit terminally ill clients to be maintained at home unless they require specialized care on a long-term basis. Some terminally ill clients are admitted to nursing facilities for care, but this would not be essential. Rather, it reflects the preferences or individual needs of the client and family.

5

Legal and Ethical Concerns Related to the Elderly Client

NURSING HIGHLIGHTS

1. To offer the highest level of service to clients and reduce personal legal liability, the gerontologic nurse should know and abide by relevant state laws, institution or agency protocols, and current professional standards of practice.
2. Many gerontologic nurses are at particular legal risk because of the settings in which they work (e.g., long-term-care facilities, home care settings) and because of the special needs of the elderly population they care for.
3. Nurses should have their own malpractice insurance in addition to that provided to them by their employer.
4. The gerontologic nurse should be aware that abuse of the elderly is often misdiagnosed as an age-related disorder, such as attributing weight loss to malnutrition or relating bruising and fractures to a tendency to fall.

GLOSSARY

informed consent—voluntary granting of permission for a procedure to be performed after the nature of the procedure and its associated risks have been fully and accurately described

malpractice—failure to meet an established standard of professional care that results in physical or psychologic harm to a client

maltreatment—any behavior that involves physical, emotional, or material abuse or neglect of another person

power of attorney (POA)—a legal written document by which a competent person designates an individual to carry on the first person's affairs when he/she is unable to do so

ENHANCED OUTLINE

See text pages
_____

I. Legal issues in gerontologic nursing

A. General liability issues
   1. The nurse should be aware of situations that can create safety hazards for the elderly (e.g., damaged equipment, wet floors, supplies left in the halls) and see that they are corrected.
   2. The nurse must provide adequate supervision of employees to be sure that elderly clients receive quality care by qualified personnel and to detect immediately any evidence of abuse or neglect by a staff member.
   3. The nurse must follow the institution's policies governing use of physical and pharmacologic restraints and must *obtain a physician's order when the use of restraints is considered absolutely necessary.*
      a) The nurse should take steps to ensure a restraint-free environment.
         (1) Interact and communicate with the client in a calm, reassuring way to reduce the need for restraints.
         (2) Ask a family member to attend the client who may be prone to wandering or inadvertent self-harm.
      b) When restraints are needed and the client or family member objects to their use, the nurse should ask the person to sign a release of liability form that outlines the risks of not using restraints.
      c) When the client is restrained, the nurse must be aware that the restraints may cause injury and so should closely observe the client.

B. Informed consent

    1. The client's informed consent should be obtained for any therapeutic procedure that goes beyond routine care covered by the blanket consent form signed at the time of admission.

    2. Barriers to informed consent among the elderly include sensory impairments, which complicate the discussion of complex procedures, and wavering levels of memory and cognition, which leave the client's actual granting of consent open to question.

    3. The physician or other health care professional who is going to perform the procedure should explain the following features to the client:

        a) Risks

        b) Expected results

        c) Options

    4. Written consent is preferred to oral consent, and the form should be signed, witnessed, and dated.

    5. The nurse should be able to explain the consent form procedures to the client and should encourage the client to ask questions.

    6. The nurse should inform the physician of any signs that the client has misunderstood the discussion that preceded the granting of consent or regrets having given it.

    7. Health care providers should not encourage the client to grant or refuse consent.

    8. The client who refuses to grant consent should be asked to sign a release stating that consent is denied and that he/she understands the potential consequences of refusal.

C. Power of attorney (POA)

    1. The nurse should ensure that elderly clients are aware of the purposes and advantages of powers of attorney and encourage them to execute such documents.

        a) Power of attorney may be broad or may be limited by duties (e.g., business, financial) or time period (e.g., usually stops if person becomes incompetent).

        b) Durable power of attorney can be set up to start or extend beyond person's becoming incompetent and is recommended for all elderly people, especially those in the early stages of dementia.

        c) Power of attorney specifically for health care (which may be called medical POA, POA for health, health care proxy, or durable POA for health care) involves one person authorizing another to make health care decisions if he/she becomes unable to do so; health care providers cannot act as witnesses to this document.

    2. The nurse must be alert to possible abuses of POA by family, personal aides, and health care facility administrators.

D. Guardianship

    1. Guardianship, or conservatorship, is a court-ordered arrangement designed to appoint a person or agency to make decisions for a person who is incompetent and unable to manage his/her affairs.

         2. Guardians may make just financial or medical decisions or may take care of all affairs.

         3. Guardians are monitored by the court.

         4. The nurse should be aware of the proper techniques to assess competence, including evaluating the person's cognitive skills, judgment, and communication skills.

         5. The nurse should know who is permitted to act legally for an incompetent person in order to avoid legal liability.

         6. The nurse should know the law concerning guardianship so that she/he may help the client, or the family of a person whose competency is suspect, reach a decision about legal guardianship.

         7. The nurse and other health care professionals should be alert to anyone seeking guardianship who may be acting out of ignorance of an older person's true status or from unethical motives.

  E. Living wills

         1. The living will (sometimes called a directive to physician or advance directive) is prepared by a competent person to advise health care personnel, family members, and clergy about that person's wishes concerning the use of extraordinary means to prolong life when an irreversible process is taking place.

         2. Copies of the living will should be on file with the client's physician and family or person who has power of attorney.

         3. The living will can be canceled by the client orally or in writing.

         4. Living wills are legally recognized in some states; rules are complex and precise and differ from state to state.

         5. The nurse must not pressure older adults into executing a living will but should help them to carry out their wishes, including obtaining legal assistance and identifying appropriate witnesses.

         6. Living wills are often not honored; the nurse should tell the client the health care facility's policy on carrying out such wishes.

  F. Wills and estate planning

         1. The nurse should suggest that the client who wishes to make a will obtain the services of a qualified attorney.

         2. The nurse should know the policies of the employing institution or agency before agreeing to witness a will for a client.

See text pages

II. Ethical issues in gerontologic nursing

  A. Ethics in gerontologic nursing practice

         1. Ethics sets forth guidelines that the nurse uses when resolving complicated situations that involve the welfare of clients.

2. An important guide to the ethical conduct of nurses is the Code for Nurses developed by the American Nurses' Association (ANA). The code upholds the dignity of all persons and emphasizes the nurse's responsibilities to protect clients from inappropriate interventions, to make appropriate nursing judgments, and to maintain professional competence and knowledge.

B. Protecting the rights of the impaired elderly
   1. Advise the client of the Patient's or Resident's Bill of Rights.
   2. Advise the client of the Patient Self-Determination Act, which requires Medicare-participating institutions to inform clients of their right to take part in decisions relating to their care.
   3. Ascertain whether the client has executed a living will (see section I,E of this chapter).
   4. Notify the client about the institution's policy relevant to honoring living wills and other directives.
   5. Determine whether there is a person holding power of attorney or functioning as a legal guardian who can make medical decisions for the impaired client (see sections I,C and I,D of this chapter).
   6. For a client assessed as incompetent who has no known support system, seek guidance from the appropriate state agency so that a guardian can be appointed by the court to make medical decisions on the client's behalf.
   7. Be sure that no procedure is done without the consent of the client or designated agent (see section I,B of this chapter).
   8. Respect the privacy and preserve the dignity of the client.

C. Principles of advocacy
   1. Gerontologic nurses are often in the position of acting to protect the rights of elderly clients.
   2. Advocates are not neutral.
   3. Areas in which nurses may act as advocates include:
      a) Improving level and quality of care for the institutionalized elderly client
      b) Finding appropriate social services for the client
   4. Advocates may represent the elderly client within their own institution, to other institutions and agencies, or to the client's family, legislators, courts, or community representatives.
   5. Advocates follow certain procedures to be effective.
      a) They have specific facts relevant to the case.
      b) They know relevant institutional policies.
      c) They know risks (e.g., losing one's job, alienating supervisors and coworkers).
      d) They are tolerant of opposing ideas and open to alternative solutions.

See text pages
_____

III. Elder abuse and neglect

A. Types of abuse
   1. Physical abuse: direct, nonaccidental physical or sexual assaults that cause bodily harm
   2. Physical neglect: passive or active failure to provide even minimally for physical safety or to prevent physical harm
   3. Psychologic abuse: direct infliction of emotional pain or the use of manipulation and coercion
   4. Psychologic neglect: passive or active failure to meet even minimally emotional needs or to provide a sense of security
   5. Exploitation: direct, nonaccidental infliction of financial or material loss through improper use of property or through failure to manage and protect property and valuables

B. Profile of abusers and victims
   1. General characteristics of abusers: There are discrepancies among research studies concerning the profile descriptions of those who abuse the elderly; the following are just selected samples.
      a) In the family: middle-aged relative of the victim; caregiver who exhibits fatigue, stress, frailty, or ignorance; person who has a poor relationship with the victim; person with a history of financial dependence on the victim; person with a history of substance abuse; person who as a child was abused by a now elderly relative
      b) In an institutional setting
         (1) Facility characteristics: for-profit status, custodial orientation, inadequate supervision, understaffing
         (2) Staff characteristics: person under great personal stress, person with negative attitude toward older adults, inexperienced staff member, person with limited education, staff member who is suffering burnout, substance abuser, person with poor coping abilities
   2. Usual characteristics of victims: female over 60, male over 75, financially dependent, significantly impaired physically and/or mentally, completely dependent on and/or loyal to the abuser, socially isolated, passive, history of a poor relationship with the abuser

C. Signs of physical abuse and neglect
   1. Signs of physical abuse: welts; multiple bruises, especially when they are in various stages of healing; genital or breast bruising or trauma; fractures, dislocations, or sprains; abrasions or lacerations in various stages of healing; injuries of the head or face, including orbital

fractures, black eyes, broken teeth, and erratic alopecia; multiple burns; human bite marks; expressions of fear, nervousness, depression, anger, emotional lability, passivity

  2. Signs of physical neglect: malnutrition, dehydration, poor hygiene, inappropriate clothing, broken assistive devices or lack of necessary devices, incontinence, fecal impaction, decayed teeth, oral thrush, pressure ulcers, contractures, hypothermia, hyperthermia, unexplained delay in seeking treatment, signs of overmedication or undermedication

D. Signs of psychologic abuse and neglect

  1. Signs of psychologic abuse: guardedness toward or clinging to the abuser, paranoia, conflicting interactions with the abuser, expression of ambivalence toward caregivers, erratic or inconsistent explanation of injuries, depression, confusion, disorientation, anger, evidence of social or physical isolation, threatening behavior displayed by the abuser

  2. Signs of psychologic neglect: clinging to a health care professional, history of limited socialization, depression, withdrawal, confusion, disorientation, anger, low self-esteem, limited interaction between the victim and the abuser, abuser speaking for the victim and not consulting the victim about his/her wishes

E. The role of the nurse in reporting suspected abuse and neglect

  1. Assess suspected victims through interviews and examination for signs of physical and psychologic abuse and neglect (see Nurse Alert, "Interviewing Possible Victims of Elder Abuse").

! NURSE *ALERT* !

Interviewing Possible Victims of Elder Abuse

Because of the physical and emotional vulnerability of the elderly people who are at high risk for abuse and neglect, the process of interviewing them requires great skill and sensitivity. The following guidelines may be helpful in speaking with possible victims.

- Conduct the interview in a private place.
- Remain calm and nonjudgmental.
- Bear in mind that the victim may be less candid if the abuser brought him/her to the interview or is waiting nearby.
- Interview the victim and abuser separately and together. Ask both to describe a typical day, listening for inconsistencies.
- Determine whether the characteristics of the victim and abuser fit established profiles (e.g., abnormal dependency, social isolation).
- Use both open-ended and specific questions about abuse and neglect and the victim's relationship with the abuser. Ask the victim for specific details about the maltreatment experienced.

2. Assess suspected abusers cautiously, being alert for signs of impulsive, destructive, or aggressive behavior. Attempt to develop a bond of trust with the abuser.
3. Determine the dangerousness of the situation and the degree of potential risk to the victim. Be particularly watchful of an abuser who displays extreme psychopathology, refusal of outside help, escalation of incidents of maltreatment, and signs of chronic rather than acute abuse.
4. Conduct a comprehensive home assessment, noting overall cleanliness; safety hazards; accessibility; overcrowding; physical signs that restraints have been used; adequacy of space and privacy for older adult; and condition, number, and appropriateness of the older adult's possessions.
5. Undertake interventions to treat the immediate effects of the maltreatment and minimize the trauma.
   a) Report elder abuse to protective agencies and abuse registries; know state laws regarding the requirements for reporting suspected or known abuse and know the definitions of types of abuse.
   b) Use crisis intervention strategies to deal with the immediate situation of abuse.
   c) Provide emergency medical treatment, shelters, financial assistance, counseling, protective services, home health care, and/or public guardianship for victims; involve the victim in the decision if possible.
6. Undertake interventions to prevent further abuse.
   a) Provide home health care services for the victim, and notify family about meal and transportation services.
   b) Provide opportunities for socialization for the victim, such as day care programs.
   c) Provide individual counseling for the victim and abuser, marital counseling, family counseling, and support groups.

See text pages

_____

IV. End-of-life issues

A. Resuscitation decisions
   1. Issues affecting decisions relevant to resuscitation orders include benefit to the client, cost of the procedure, availability of resources, trauma to the client, seriousness of the illness, and quality of life that can be reached; age should not be a factor.
   2. Unless a medical order specifically states that a client is not to be resuscitated (a no-code or do-not-resuscitate [DNR] order), failing to attempt to do so could be regarded as negligence.

3. The nurse should withdraw from a client's case if she/he is not able to honor the client's wishes.
4. No-code orders must be placed on the physician's order sheet and signed.
    a) The placement of a special no-code symbol by the client's bed or the insertion of "DNR" on the care plan is not legal if there is no physician's order.
    b) Advance directives cannot be honored until appropriate physician's orders are written.
5. Consent for the no-code decision should be obtained from the client if possible or from the family or legal guardian.
6. The nurse must abide by the specific policies of the agency or institution regarding no-code orders.

B. Euthanasia
    1. Passive euthanasia
        a) In passive euthanasia, no medical assistance or extraordinary means are used to prolong the life of a person who is near death as the result of old age or severe illness; only comfort and supportive measures are given.
        b) A decision in favor of passive euthanasia should be made by the client and/or family.
        c) The members of the health care team should not play an active role in the choice of passive euthanasia.
        d) Serious ethical concerns and legal liability arise about removing life-sustaining equipment.
    2. Active euthanasia
        a) In active euthanasia (e.g., assisted suicide), a client requests that life be ended by another person by a means that assures that death will occur.
        b) Active euthanasia is illegal.

C. Nursing considerations associated with caring for dying clients
    1. To help the dying client, you must first resolve your own feelings about death.
    2. The care offered to a dying client must be comfort-oriented, not cure-oriented; keep the client clean, dry, and free of pain.
    3. Control the client's physical pain on the basis of his/her report of its severity; also continually assess for signs of discomfort because the elderly client may deny the presence of pain.
    4. Manage respiratory distress by maintaining a calm atmosphere, positioning the client to achieve maximum ventilation, and administering sedatives cautiously and oxygen if needed.
    5. Assist the client in maintaining his/her appearance.
    6. Encourage the client to continue to make his/her own decisions.
    7. Respect the client's desire for togetherness or privacy, and encourage the family to abide by his/her wishes.
    8. Discourage the family and staff from talking about the client in his/her presence if the client is not included in the conversation.

9. Encourage the client to share feelings about death and to express preferences about the way he/she wishes to die. Respect those preferences as faithfully as possible.
10. Help the client look beyond his/her present debility and focus on the ways that life has been useful, productive, and happy.
11. Encourage the client to undertake a life review and recall happy incidents from the past.
12. Provide support to the client's family during the dying process and after death.
13. Evaluate the client's death, considering the level of comfort, cleanliness, control, and fear that was experienced.

1. Mr. Jenner, a resident in a long-term-care facility, has repeatedly attempted to leave through the back door. The nurse catches him attempting to leave for the third time in 1 day and says, "If you do that one more time, I'm going to have to tie you up in a chair!" The nurse could be found guilty of:

   a. Assault.
   b. Battery.
   c. False imprisonment.
   d. Malpractice.

2. Which of the following is most likely to invalidate a client's informed consent for surgery?

   a. The nurse answers questions about the procedure after the client has signed the consent form.
   b. The nurse discovers that the client could not read the fine print on the consent form the client signed.
   c. The nurse notifies the physician that the client has misconceptions about the procedure.
   d. The client received meperidine (Demerol) for pain 8 hours prior to signing the consent form.

3. An elderly client tells the nurse that she would like her youngest son to make health care decisions for her if she becomes incompetent. The nurse should suggest that she have her son:

   a. Assigned as executor.
   b. Appointed as guardian.
   c. Appointed as conservator.
   d. Given power of attorney (POA).

4. Mr. Stein is admitted to the hospital in a state that legally recognizes living wills. He is comatose and his daughter has his power of attorney. Which of the following takes legal precedence in determining whether Mr. Stein will be resuscitated if he stops breathing?

   a. Mr. Stein's living will
   b. The daughter's wishes

   c. The physician's orders
   d. Hospital policies

5. Which of the following nurses is applying the ethical principle of beneficence?

   a. A nurse who disguises the client's anti-hypertensive medication in food after the client refuses to take it
   b. A nurse who spends an equal amount of time with each of his/her assigned clients
   c. A nurse who questions the physician's order for tube feedings based on knowledge of the client's desire to avoid invasive measures
   d. A nurse who assists the client's family to access resources that will permit them to care for the client at home

6. Which of the following nursing actions is based on provisions of the American Nurses' Association (ANA) Code of Ethics?

   a. Preparing a written nursing care plan for each client
   b. Teaching the family to perform some of the client's treatments
   c. Refusing to carry out an inappropriate medical order
   d. Encouraging elderly clients to participate in research about nursing care

7. Ms. Devlin is terminally ill and unable to speak for herself. Her daughter has been asked to decide whether to have intravenous (IV) fluids started for Ms. Devlin. The nurse encourages the daughter to make the choice that the daughter believes she can be most comfortable with. This nurse is applying which ethical philosophy?

   a. Utilitarian
   b. Egoistic
   c. Relativistic
   d. Naturalistic

8. Which of the following assessments suggests that an elderly client is a victim of physical abuse?

   a. Multiple petechiae on the legs
   b. Contractures of the extremities
   c. Clinging to the caregiving family member
   d. Ecchymotic areas on the arms and shoulders

9. Which of the following reflects the best technique when interviewing a suspected victim of elder abuse?

   a. Ask another health care professional to be present to verify observations.
   b. Have the caregiver wait outside the room during the interview.
   c. Avoid expressing negative responses toward the abuser.
   d. Avoid asking for specific details about abusive actions.

10. Which of the following is most likely to be cited by the abuser of an elderly person as the reason for the abuse?

    a. The elderly person is very dependent on the abuser.
    b. The elderly person controls the abuser's behavior by withholding financial resources.
    c. The elderly person continues to make his/her own decisions despite needing help with care.
    d. The abuser feels responsible for control of the elderly person's behavior.

11. Extraordinary measures in the treatment of a terminally ill client would include:

    a. Feedings by gastrostomy tube.
    b. Oxygen by nasal cannula.
    c. Intramuscular injections of antibiotics.
    d. Intravenous (IV) infusion of narcotics.

12. Which of the following reflects the most appropriate action for a nurse to take if he/she disagrees with a client's decision to refuse measures to prolong life?

    a. Consult with the physician about ordering appropriate measures to enhance the client's life.

    b. Notify the hospital's ethics committee of his/her concerns regarding the client's decision.
    c. Contact his/her supervisor to request not to be assigned to this client's care.
    d. Meet with the client and family to discuss his/her concerns about the client's decision.

ANSWERS

1. **Correct answer is a.** The nurse has threatened to tie Mr. Jenner to a chair. If Mr. Jenner perceives this as a threat of harm or as keeping him confined against his will, the nurse may be guilty of assault.

   b. Battery is touching without consent. The nurse has not touched Mr. Jenner.
   c. If the nurse actually ties Mr. Jenner to a chair without an order for that form of restraint, it may be false imprisonment.
   d. Malpractice requires failure to meet an established standard of care that results in physical or psychologic harm to the client. Since no harm to Mr. Jenner is apparent, malpractice has not occurred.

2. **Correct answer is b.** Sensory deficits, such as poor vision or deafness, that prevent the client from understanding the information that is provided about a surgical procedure may invalidate the consent. In this case, the client could not read the printed description of the procedure and its complications; therefore, the consent may not be informed.

   a. It is the responsibility of the nurse to continue to answer questions and reinforce explanations even after the client has consented. If the client later expresses a desire to revoke consent, the nurse should notify the physician.
   c. This action is appropriate and does not necessarily invalidate the consent. The physician may need to explain the procedure further and confirm the consent. If the

physician takes no action, the nurse should notify his/her superior of the client's misconceptions before allowing the procedure to be performed.

d. Demerol has a short half-life and would not be expected to still be acting 8 hours after administration.

3. **Correct answer is d.** Giving her son power of attorney specifically for health care will give him the legal right to make health care decisions for her if she is incapacitated.

   a. An executor is appointed to oversee the carrying out of the person's wishes as expressed in a will. The appointment becomes effective only after death.
   b. A guardian is appointed by the court to legally act for a person who is legally declared incompetent.
   c. A conservator is appointed by the court to manage the affairs of a person who is mentally incompetent.

4. **Correct answer is c.** The physician's orders ultimately determine the care to be provided. Most physicians will be guided by a client's stated wishes in a living will and/or by the wishes of the person with power of attorney.

   a. The living will does not carry legal weight until a physician's order is written covering its provisions.
   b. The wishes of the person with power of attorney provide guidance to the physician with regard to no-code orders, but the order must be written by the physician.
   d. In states whose laws give legal weight to living wills, hospital policy cannot deny the client the right to refuse resuscitative measures.

5. **Correct answer is a.** Disguising medication in food reflects the assumption that the nurse, because of professional education and awareness of research, knows what is best for the client (the principle of beneficence).

   b. This nurse is applying the principle of justice by equally distributing the benefits of his/her care.

c. This nurse is applying the principle of autonomy by advocating the client's right to make his/her own choice.
d. This nurse is applying the principle of family responsibility, which assumes that families are obligated to care for their own members.

6. **Correct answer is c.** The ANA Code of Ethics indicates that the nurse has an obligation to safeguard the client from incompetent practice by any individual.

   a and b. The ANA Code of Ethics does not address the methodology for care planning or family participation in care.
   d. Although the ANA Code of Ethics does promote the individual nurse's participation in activities that contribute to development of nursing knowledge, it also includes provisions that address respect for clients' rights. Clients must be permitted to make their own decisions about participation in research. The nurse's encouragement could be perceived by the client as indicating that quality of care depends on participating in the research, which would be coercive.

7. **Correct answer is d.** The naturalist identifies good as that which produces positive attitudes or interests.

   a. The utilitarian sees the good as that from which the greatest number of people benefit.
   b. The egoist proposes that an act which provides the greatest benefit to oneself is morally correct.
   c. The relativist applies the overall beliefs of society at a given time to determine what is good.

8. **Correct answer is d.** Ecchymoses, or bruises, on the arms and shoulders may indicate rough handling by the caregiver.

   a. Petechiae are seldom related to trauma. They are more likely related to nutritional deficits or medication effects.
   b. Contractures are the result of physical neglect, not abuse.

c. Clinging to an abuser is more likely a sign of psychologic abuse. An elderly client who is fearful of new surroundings may also cling to the usual caregiver.

9. **Correct answer is c.** The interviewer must remain calm and nonjudgmental. The victim of abuse often has ambivalent feelings about the abuser. If the nurse expresses negative responses to the abuser, the victim may respond defensively.

   a. Privacy is important to permit the victim to feel comfortable disclosing the abuse. The presence of additional personnel may discourage honest revelations.
   b. The victim may be less candid if he/she is aware that the abuser is waiting nearby.
   d. It is important to ask both open-ended and specific questions. Specific details of the abuse are necessary to permit appropriate interventions.

10. **Correct answer is b.** Abusers often indicate that manipulation by the elderly person, through withholding approval, appreciation, or financial resources, has motivated the abuse.

    a. This may be a result of the abusive relationship but is not usually offered as a reason for the abuse.
    c. The elderly person who remains autonomous is less likely to be abused than a confused person who cannot provide any of his/her own care.
    d. By itself, feeling responsible for the older person's behavior does not produce abuse. If the caregiver feels embarrassed or frustrated by an inability to control the older

person's behavior, the potential for abuse increases.

11. **Correct answer is a.** Extraordinary measures are those which do not offer hope for reversal of the terminal condition but cause expense, pain, or high risk for complications. Because insertion of a gastrostomy tube is a surgical procedure and can be very expensive, it can be considered an extraordinary measure.

    b. Oxygen may relieve dyspnea and is not unreasonably expensive, so it is considered an ordinary measure.
    c. Because antibiotics are curative for infections, they are not considered extraordinary measures, despite the pain of the injections and the potential expense of the drugs.
    d. Because the pain control achieved with narcotics may contribute greatly to quality of life, even IV administration may be considered a comfort measure.

12. **Correct answer is c.** The nurse who feels unable to follow the client's expressed wishes should request to be removed from the case.

    a. It would be inappropriate to ask the physician to order care based on the nurse's wishes rather than those of the family or client.
    b. The ethics committee would appropriately be involved in decisions to terminate life-sustaining treatments, not in the client's decision about refusing such care.
    d. It is inappropriate and unethical for the nurse to encourage the client to follow any particular course of action.

6

Cardiovascular and Peripheral Vascular Disorders

NURSING HIGHLIGHTS

1. The elderly are at increased risk for many cardiovascular disorders, such as congestive heart failure and hypertension.
2. Nurses are often in the best position to learn that a client is experiencing 1 or more warning signs of a cerebrovascular accident (CVA), and prompt intervention may prevent serious disability or death.
3. When assessing cardiovascular status, the nurse should pay particular attention to the client's breathing pattern. Acute dyspnea can be a symptom of myocardial infarction (MI) in older adults and requires immediate medical attention.
4. Myocardial infarction is often misdiagnosed or diagnosed after a significant delay in older clients because the elderly often experience less pain at the time of the MI than do younger persons.

GLOSSARY

drop attack—a fall caused by muscular flaccidity in the legs that is not accompanied by altered consciousness

hemianopia—blindness or impaired vision in half the visual field of one or both eyes

intermittent claudication—leg pain that occurs during walking or other exercise due to decreased blood flow; relieved by rest

intima—the innermost layer of a structure, especially of a blood vessel

parenchyma—the tissue of an organ

rest pain—burning pain caused by ischemia of nerves when arterial blood flow to legs is inadequate; occurs at rest when legs are elevated and is relieved when legs are dependent

vasopressor—a drug that constricts the blood vessels, especially the arteries and arterioles

ENHANCED OUTLINE

I. Cardiovascular disorders

See text pages

_____

A. Age-related changes (see section II,A of Chapter 2)

B. General nursing assessment
   1. General observation
      a) Observe the client's activity tolerance.
      b) Assess the client's breathing pattern while the client is walking, sitting down or standing up, and talking.
      c) Note the client's overall coloring; pallor may be a sign of cardiovascular disorders.
      d) Assess color of mucous membranes, lips, and nipples.
      e) Observe the condition of the nails and nail beds.
         (1) Assess capillary refill time by checking how fast the fingernail returns to pink after sufficient pressure is applied to the nail to make the skin under it turn white; delayed capillary refill time may be a sign of cardiovascular disease.
         (2) Check for the presence of clubbing (see Figures 2-1 and 2-2 in Chapter 2).
      f) Inspect the ankles and fingers for the presence of edema.
      g) Inspect the vessels and skin on the head, neck, and extremities for varicosities, redness, and jugular vein distention.
      h) Note the amount and distribution of hair on the extremities; hair loss may be associated with impaired circulation.
      i) Check level of consciousness and cognitive function, noting any signs of confusion.
   2. Interview
      a) Ask the client about factors that may contribute to the development of cardiovascular disease (e.g., family history, high intake of calories, salt, and animal fat; obesity; smoking; lack of exercise; sustained stress; internalizing of emotions).

b) Inquire about current or past disorders that may affect cardiovascular function (e.g., diabetes, hypoglycemia, hypertension, anemia, malnutrition, renal disorders, infections, pneumonia, surgeries).

c) Inquire about the presence of symptoms of cardiovascular disease (e.g., fatigue; lightheadedness; dizziness; palpitations; breathing difficulties; blackouts; edema; cold extremities; chest pain or pressure; unusual sensations in chest, back, neck, arms, or jaws).

d) Ask if the client or family member has noticed any recent changes in physical or mental function.

e) Ask whether the client is allergic to iodine or seafood; diagnostic procedures may involve the injection of radiopaque dyes that contain iodine.

3. Physical examination
   a) Check the extremities.
      (1) Presence of edema
      (2) Temperature
      (3) Distribution of hair
   b) Assess radial, apical, and pedal pulses.
   c) Check for postural hypotension by assessing blood pressure in 3 different positions (sitting, standing, and supine); provide safety measures in case of a fall.
   d) Auscultate the heart and palpate the point of maximal impulse (the area on the chest where the apex beat of the heart is detected).

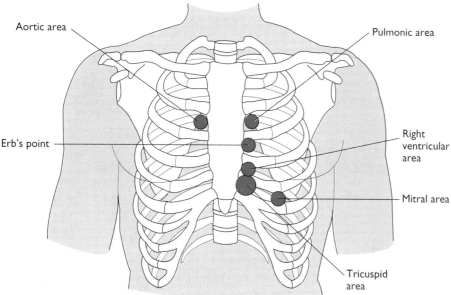

Figure 6–1
Areas for Myocardial Assessment

C. Common disorders
  1. Hypertension
     a) Definition: persistently high (on 3 separate occasions) arterial blood pressure (160/95 mm Hg in age 65 and over); increased incidence with age

     b) Pathophysiology and etiology
        (1) Pathophysiology: a disorder or imbalance in the control systems that regulate blood pressure (arterial baroceptor system, renin-angiotensin system, vascular autoregulation, and body fluid volume)
        (2) Etiology
           (a) Essential (primary or idiopathic) hypertension: genetic predisposition, excessive dietary salt intake, alterations in sodium metabolism
           (b) Secondary hypertension: renal vascular or parenchymal disease, arteriosclerosis, atherosclerosis, hyperthyroidism, Paget's disease, endocrine disorders, anemia, parkinsonism, brain tumors, thiamine deficiency, psychiatric disturbances
     c) Symptoms: *usually asymptomatic in the elderly until severe or until complications develop;* when seen, dull headache at waking, slow tremor, epistaxis, disorientation, confusion, memory loss
     d) Treatment: rest; reduced sodium intake; weight reduction (when appropriate); smoking cessation; reduced alcohol intake; effective management of stressors; antihypertensive therapy; careful monitoring for signs of drug-related hypotension (e.g., dizziness, syncope, restlessness, drowsiness), which may occur in the elderly when blood pressure of 190/100 mm Hg drops to 140/70 mm Hg
  2. Congestive heart failure
     a) Definition: inability of the heart to maintain adequate cardiac output; increased incidence and prevalence with age
     b) Pathophysiology and etiology
        (1) Pathophysiology: alterations of basic cardiac mechanisms, such as heart rate, stroke volume, cardiac output, preload, afterload, and contractility, leading to failure to empty venous reservoirs and reduced delivery of blood into arterial circulation
        (2) Etiology
           (a) Conditions: hypertension, coronary artery disease, mitral valve stenosis, cor pulmonale, subacute bacterial endocarditis, pneumonia, pulmonary emboli, anemia, congenital heart disease, renal disease, liver disease, hyperthyroidism, chronic obstructive pulmonary disease (COPD)

(b) Associations among the elderly: too much or too little activity; emotional stress; some cardiac drugs (e.g., disopyramide, steroids)

c) Symptoms: *may be obscured by other diseases in the elderly;* when seen, weakness, fatigue, confusion, agitation, insomnia, depression, nighttime wandering

d) Treatment: partial or total bed rest; administration of digitalis (see Client Teaching Checklist, "Signs of Digitalis Toxicity"), diuretics, and vasodilators; oxygen therapy; reduced sodium intake; meticulous skin care; changes in positioning; emotional support

3. Cerebrovascular accident (CVA)

   a) Definition: a disruption of the brain's normal blood supply; increased risk with age

   b) Pathophysiology and etiology

      (1) Pathophysiology: partial or complete cerebral thrombosis, embolus lodging in cerebral vessels, ruptured cerebral blood vessel (not common)

      (2) Etiology: hypertension, atherosclerosis, arteriosclerosis, dehydration, glucose intolerance, silent myocardial infarction, mitral stenosis, prolonged atrial fibrillation, anemia, high serum triglyceride level

   c) Symptoms (may be subtle): headache, lightheadedness, numbness, tingling, dizziness, drop attack, memory impairment, behavioral changes, hemiplegia, aphasia, hemianopia

---

✔ CLIENT TEACHING CHECKLIST ✔

Signs of Digitalis Toxicity

Emphasize the importance of the client's reporting the following signs and symptoms of digitalis toxicity:

✔ Disorientation or confusion (often the earliest sign in the elderly)

✔ Headache

✔ Restlessness or irritability

✔ Lassitude or depression

✔ Visual disturbances, most commonly halos around objects and shimmering visual field

✔ Anorexia

✔ Nausea, vomiting, or diarrhea

✔ Abdominal pain

✔ Bradycardia

      d) Treatment: administration of anticoagulant therapy (in cerebral thrombosis and emboli), osmotic diuretics, or thrombolytic enzymes; surgical intervention; rehabilitation

4. Pulmonary embolism
   a) Definition: obstruction of the pulmonary artery or 1 of its branches by a blood clot or other substance; may cause death instantaneously
   b) Pathophysiology and etiology
      (1) Pathophysiology: passage of venous clots from the lower extremities, pelvis, or the endocardium of the right ventricle following myocardial infarction
      (2) Etiology: congestive heart failure, recent surgery, hip fracture, arrhythmia, history of thrombosis, malnutrition, immobility, debilitating disease
   c) Symptoms
      (1) Small area of lung infarction: tachycardia, dyspnea, pain, low-grade fever, cough, bloody sputum
      (2) Large area of lung infarction: severe dyspnea and pain, tachycardia, cyanosis, shock
   d) Treatment: bed rest, control of hypotension with vasopressors, oxygen therapy, administration of analgesics and intravenous heparin, pulmonary embolectomy, insertion of umbrella filter in vena cava, application of clips to the inferior vena cava

5. Myocardial infarction (MI)
   a) Definition: necrosis of the myocardium as a result of a decrease in the supply of oxygenated blood from the coronary arteries
   b) Pathophysiology and etiology
      (1) Pathophysiology: formation of a thrombus in the coronary artery, contributing to the interruption of blood flow to the myocardium, followed by infarction, or necrosis, of the heart muscle
      (2) Etiology: atherosclerotic coronary artery disease, hypertension
   c) Symptoms: acute dyspnea; pain, which may be less severe in the elderly, that may radiate to the left arm, chest, neck, and abdomen; pallor; sweating; decreased blood pressure; rapid, weak pulse; slight fever; elevated sedimentation rate; anuria; arrhythmia; apprehension
   d) Treatment: bed and armchair rest; drug therapy: thrombolytics, anticoagulants, antiarrhythmics, analgesics, and tranquilizers; close monitoring for internal bleeding, pulmonary edema, venous thrombosis, pulmonary or arterial embolism, congestive heart failure, arrhythmia, and cardiogenic shock

D. Essential nursing care
   1. Nursing assessment (same as section I,B of this chapter)
   2. Nursing diagnoses
      a) Pain related to impaired coronary blood flow
      b) Altered cardiopulmonary tissue perfusion related to decreased cardiac output
      c) Activity intolerance related to inadequate oxygen supply to tissues
      d) Impaired verbal communication related to dysphasia
      e) Impaired physical mobility related to hemiplegia
      f) Fluid volume excess related to decreased cardiac output
      g) Altered nutrition, less than body requirements, related to nonacceptance of prescribed diet
      h) Anxiety related to fear of unknown procedures, death
   3. Nursing implementation (intervention)
      a) Administer analgesics and oxygen as prescribed.
      b) Document and report signs of impaired tissue perfusion, including hypotension, tachycardia, and disorientation.
      c) Teach the client exercises that will safely increase activity tolerance.
      d) Establish an alternative means of communicating with a client who has had a cerebrovascular accident, such as use of a picture board.
      e) Turn the client frequently to prevent skin breakdown.
      f) Reinforce teaching given by physical therapist; check understanding and compliance.
      g) Encourage the client to participate in activities of daily living (ADLs) to the fullest possible extent.
      h) Discuss dietary modifications that will reduce edema.
      i) Compensate for diminished appetite by serving a greater number of smaller meals throughout the day rather than 3 large ones; suggest using seasonings other than salt, which the elderly may use excessively due to decreased taste perception.
      j) Encourage the client and the client's family to discuss their concerns.
   4. Nursing evaluation
      a) The client states that pain is relieved.
      b) The client maintains blood pressure and heart rate within normal range and is oriented to person, place, and time.
      c) The client participates in an appropriate exercise program.
      d) The client's activity tolerance improves.
      e) The client uses and expresses satisfaction with alternative means of communication.
      f) The client's skin remains intact.
      g) The client participates in rehabilitation program.
      h) The client undertakes activities of daily living to the limits of his/her abilities.
      i) The client is free from edema.

      j) The client maintains an adequate intake of appropriate foods.

      k) The client and family state that they feel less anxious.

5. Gerontologic nursing considerations

    a) Dietary changes and other nondrug therapy may be preferred to antihypertensive drug therapy as the latter may lead to sudden decreases in blood pressure due to cerebral or coronary insufficiency in older adults.

    b) The elderly have an increased chance of experiencing adverse reactions to antihypertensive medication.

    c) Be aware of noncompliance issues related to antihypertensive medications, especially that the client who is feeling better or who is experiencing adverse side effects may stop taking the medication.

    d) Elderly clients with congestive heart failure have reduced cardiac reserve, increased risk of skin breakdown, and increased risk of complications associated with immobility (e.g., pneumonia, pulmonary embolism).

    e) For the elderly client who has experienced a cerebrovascular accident (CVA), the emphasis is on rehabilitation. Gather accurate data about person's functioning level before the stroke (e.g., memory), and set rehabilitation goals that the client accepts as realistic.

    f) Testing for isoenzymes of creatine kinase (CK) and lactate dehydrogenase (LDH) is particularly important in detecting myocardial infarction (MI) in the elderly, who may have few symptoms; levels of CK and LDH may not be as significantly elevated as in younger clients.

II. Peripheral vascular disorders

> See text pages
> _____

A. Age-related changes (see section II,A of Chapter 2)

B. General nursing assessment

1. General observation

    a) Observe the client for signs of peripheral vascular disorders, including slow gait, rubbing the legs, or removing shoes.

    b) Check the client's extremities for edema, varicosities, discoloration, and sores.

2. Interview

    a) Ask the client about risk factors for peripheral vascular disorders (e.g., inappropriate diet, smoking, lack of exercise, wearing of constricting clothing, habitual crossing of legs, occupations that require long periods of standing or sitting).

b) Ask the client about the following signs or symptoms of peripheral vascular disease: cold or numb extremities; scaling of skin on the extremities; pain, fatigue, or swelling in legs after standing or walking; dark spots or sores on legs; and periods of confusion, lightheadedness, or dizziness.

c) Inquire about any family history of peripheral vascular disease.

3. Physical examination

a) Palpate the following pulses for rhythm, rate, quality, contour, and equality: temporal, brachial, radial, ulnar, femoral, popliteal, posterior tibial, and dorsalis pedis.

b) Inspect legs for signs of phlebitis, including edema, redness, tenderness, and pain in the calf on dorsiflexion of the foot (positive Homans' sign).

c) Examine the legs for edema, scaling skin, discoloration, pallor, tortuous veins, and hair loss.

d) Evaluate the skin temperature of the extremities by touching the surface of the skin at various points.

e) Check the nails for abnormal thickness, dryness, and clubbing.

C. Common disorders

1. Arteriosclerosis

a) Definition: thickening and loss of elasticity of arterial walls, often affecting the smaller vessels farthest from the heart

b) Pathophysiology and etiology

(1) Pathophysiology: fibromuscular or endothelial thickening of the walls of small arteries and arterioles

(2) Etiology: hypertension, consumption of excessive dietary fat, inadequate fiber intake, elevated serum cholesterol and triglyceride levels, obesity, smoking, lack of exercise, sustained stress, diabetes, gout

c) Symptoms: pain; dry skin; hair loss on the extremities; finger clubbing; pallor; discolorations on extremities; bruits in the carotid, aortic, femoral, or popliteal arteries; temperature differences in the lower extremities; changes in pulse intensity

d) Treatment: limitation of dietary fat and cholesterol; increased consumption of dietary fiber; weight reduction; elimination of smoking; adoption of exercise program; administration of vasodilators, antihypertensives, and cholesterol-lowering drugs; sympathetic ganglionectomy; client education about Buerger-Allen exercises and care of the feet and legs (see Client Teaching Checklist, "Foot and Leg Care for Clients with Peripheral Vascular Disorders")

2. Arteriosclerosis obliterans (thromboangiitis obliterans, Buerger's disease)

a) Definition: complete blockage of the lumen of an artery due to proliferation of the intima of the small vessels, resulting in ischemic lesions in extremities of the elderly

    b) Pathophysiology and etiology
       (1) Pathophysiology: inflammation of the small arteries and veins of the extremities, resulting in thrombus formation and vessel occlusion
       (2) Etiology: heavy smoking, diabetes, emotional stress
    c) Symptoms: rest pain (in late stages), intermittent claudication, feeling of coldness in the extremities, sensitivity to cold, redness or cyanosis, superficial thrombophlebitis, neuropathy, paresthesia, decreased or absent pulses, dermal ulcers, gangrene, sepsis

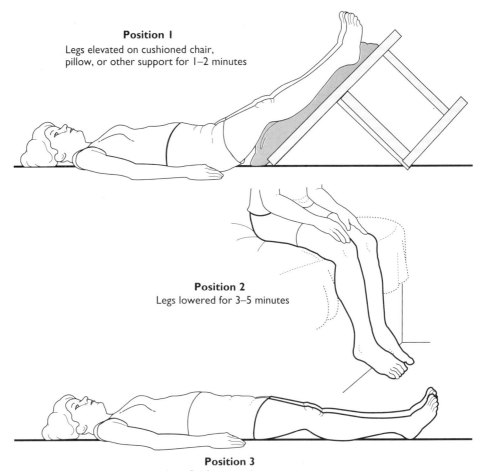

Position 1
Legs elevated on cushioned chair, pillow, or other support for 1–2 minutes

Position 2
Legs lowered for 3–5 minutes

Position 3
Legs flat for several minutes

3 positions repeated 5–6 times, 3–4 times a day

Figure 6–2
Buerger-Allen Exercises

Foot and Leg Care for Clients with Peripheral Vascular Disorder

Because even minor foot and leg injuries can lead to limb-threatening conditions in older persons with peripheral vascular disorders, discuss the following guidelines with clients:

✔ Wash feet daily with warm water and mild soap and blot them dry; be especially careful to dry the skin between the toes.

✔ Do not expose feet and legs to extremes of cold or heat; avoid sunburn.

✔ Avoid traumatic injury to feet by never going barefoot, exercising caution in crowded areas, cutting toenails carefully, and consulting a podiatrist about the management of corns, calluses, blisters, and ingrown toenails.

✔ Wear comfortable shoes that provide adequate support.

✔ Avoid clothing that constricts the blood vessels of the legs, such as socks or knee-high stockings with tight elastic bands.

✔ Do not cross the legs at the knees.

✔ Examine feet and legs daily for redness or other discoloration, cuts, or other signs of injury and report them to the physician at once.

d) Treatment: elimination of smoking, stress reduction, protection of extremities from infection and trauma, regional sympathetic block, ganglionectomy, amputation

3. Peripheral vascular disorders associated with diabetes
   a) Definition: diabetes-associated neuropathies and infections that may affect vessels throughout the body
   b) Pathophysiology and etiology
      (1) Pathophysiology: atherosclerotic changes in large blood vessels of the lower extremities, leading to occlusive peripheral arterial disease
      (2) Etiology: diabetes of several years' duration, especially when blood glucose levels have been poorly controlled
   c) Symptoms: rest pain, intermittent claudication, arterial pulses that are absent or difficult to find, skin discoloration, ulcers, gangrene, loss of pedal sensation
   d) Treatment: dietary management of obesity, hyperlipidemia, and hypertension; blood glucose control; moderate exercise, such as walking, timed to promote lowering of postmeal hyperglycemia; administration of analgesics; amputation (in severe cases)

4. Aneurysm
   a) Definition
      (1) A sac formed by the dilation of an artery or vein
      (2) Occurs most commonly in the abdominal aorta and the popliteal and femoral arteries
   b) Pathophysiology and etiology

              (1) Pathophysiology: damaged media (middle layer) in the affected blood vessel, caused by trauma, congenital weakness, or disease

              (2) Etiology: advanced arteriosclerosis, hypertension, trauma, infection, syphilis; angina pectoris, arteriosclerotic lesions, congestive heart failure, and myocardial infarction (aneurysms of the abdominal aorta)

        c) Symptoms: pain, pulsating mass that can be palpated, systolic bruit over the mass

        d) Treatment: prompt surgical intervention to prevent rupture; monitoring for postsurgical complications, including thrombus, hemorrhage, cerebral vascular accident, myocardial infarction, and acute renal insufficiency

     5. Venous thromboembolism

        a) Definition: obstruction of a vein with thrombotic material

        b) Pathophysiology and etiology

              (1) Pathophysiology: formation of an aggregate of platelets attached to the wall of the vein and a "tail" consisting of white blood cells, fibrin, and red blood cells

              (2) Etiology: immobility, fractures or surgery of the lower extremities, previous venous insufficiency, obesity

        c) Symptoms

              (1) Involvement of veins of the calf muscles: edema; warmth over affected area; pain, especially in the sole of the foot; discoloration

              (2) Involvement of inferior vena cava: bilateral edema, cyanosis and aching in lower extremities, tenderness along femoral veins, engorgement of superficial veins

              (3) Involvement of the iliofemoral segment: similar symptoms to those of inferior vena cava involvement, but occurring unilaterally

        d) Treatment: application of elastic bandages or stockings; moist heat; use of intermittent pneumatic compression (IPC) devices; elevation of affected limb; rest; avoidance of straining; sufficient hydration; administration of analgesics, anticoagulants, and thrombolytics; thrombectomy; surgical insertion of a vena cava filter

  D. Essential nursing care

     1. Nursing assessment (same as section II,B of this chapter)

     2. Nursing diagnoses

        a) Altered peripheral tissue perfusion related to impaired circulation

        b) Pain related to inadequate peripheral circulation

c) High risk for infection related to impaired circulation
d) Impaired skin integrity related to inadequate oxygen transport
e) Constipation related to restricted physical activity and drug regimen
f) High risk for injury related to altered cerebral circulation
g) Knowledge deficit related to self-care activities
h) Body image disturbance related to therapeutic amputation

3. Nursing implementation (intervention)
   a) Improve blood supply to the extremities by teaching the client to position the extremities below the level of the heart.
   b) Educate the client in pain-reduction techniques (weight control, stopping smoking, avoiding constricting clothing and leg-crossing, and doing Buerger-Allen exercises).
   c) Alert the client to the signs of and dangers associated with fungal foot infection.
   d) Teach the client to minimize the risk of venous stasis ulcers and other skin problems by avoiding injury to the extremities, particularly the feet, and avoiding tight-fitting clothing and poorly fitting shoes.
   e) Explain how to prevent constipation (adequate consumption of dietary fiber and fluids).
   f) Emphasize the necessity of complying with drug regimen and other therapeutic measures that will reduce confusion and disorientation.
   g) Provide written instructions about drug regimen, foot and leg care, and clothing restrictions.
   h) Teach the client how to prevent skin breakdown and other problems that may be associated with the use of a prosthesis.

4. Nursing evaluation
   a) The client's extremities are warm to the touch and have a normal color.
   b) The client's pain is relieved.
   c) The client uses analgesics as prescribed.
   d) The client remains free of infection.
   e) The client's skin remains intact.
   f) The client maintains normal patterns of elimination.
   g) The client remains alert and oriented to person, place, and time.
   h) The client understands the therapeutic regimen, including drug therapy, care of the extremities, and types of clothing to be avoided.
   i) The client adapts to the use of a prosthesis.

5. Gerontologic nursing consideration: Some signs of arterial insufficiency may be signs of normal aging (e.g., thickened nails, hair loss, cold feet), but these signs must be evaluated thoroughly.

1. An appropriate goal of dietary and exercise modifications for the elderly client is a serum cholesterol level below:

   a. 120 mg/dl.
   b. 170 mg/dl.
   c. 200 mg/dl.
   d. 240 mg/dl.

2. Which of the following would be considered a significant abnormality in the elderly adult?

   a. Pulse rate of 54 during sleep
   b. Blood pressure (BP) of 140/84 supine and 118/80 standing
   c. BP 154/92 at 10:00 A.M., 158/94 at 4:00 P.M., 150/90 at 10:00 P.M.
   d. Pulse rate that remains 112, 30 minutes after strenuous exercise

3. To maintain cardiovascular fitness in the bedridden elderly client, which of the following exercises would be best?

   a. Lifting 5-lb weights with both arms
   b. Isometric leg exercises
   c. Hourly position changes
   d. Passive range-of-motion exercises to arms and legs

4. The nurse should advise the elderly client with hypertension to:

   a. Reduce dietary calcium.
   b. Avoid aerobic exercise.
   c. Reduce alcohol intake.
   d. Limit fluid intake.

5. The elderly client with congestive heart failure (CHF) who is taking digitalis should be monitored for which of the following signs of toxicity?

   a. Disorientation
   b. Weight gain
   c. Constipation
   d. Dyspnea

6. An appropriate nursing diagnosis for a client who has congestive heart failure (CHF) would be:

   a. Fluid volume deficit.
   b. Impaired verbal communication.
   c. Chronic pain.
   d. Activity intolerance.

7. Eighty-year-old Mr. Wilson is beginning cardiac rehabilitation following a myocardial infarction (MI). His physician has prescribed progressively increasing aerobic exercise. To evaluate Mr. Wilson's tolerance for the exercise program, the nurse should assess for:

   a. Leg pain.
   b. Decreased blood pressure.
   c. Tachycardia.
   d. Cyanosis.

8. The nurse should advise the client who has had a cerebrovascular accident (CVA) to make which of the following dietary alterations?

   a. Reduce potassium intake.
   b. Increase fiber intake.
   c. Increase intake of vitamin K.
   d. Increase dietary protein.

9. In the early stages of arteriosclerosis obliterans, the client is most likely to complain of:

   a. Burning pain in the legs that wakens him/her at night.
   b. Numbness of the feet and ankles with exercise.
   c. Pain while walking that becomes severe enough to force him/her to stop.
   d. Increasing warmth and redness of the legs when they are elevated.

10. Treatment during the acute stage of venous thromboembolism is likely to include:

    a. Application of elastic stockings.
    b. Daily walks.

c. Passive range-of-motion exercises to the legs.

d. Use of ice packs to control pain.

11. Correct performance of Buerger-Allen exercises includes:

a. Alternately dorsiflexing and plantar flexing the feet while the legs are elevated.

b. Massaging the legs beginning at the feet and moving toward the heart.

c. Alternately walking short distances and resting with the legs elevated.

d. Elevating the legs, then dangling them, then lying flat for prescribed time periods.

12. Appropriate foot care for the client with a peripheral vascular disorder includes:

a. Soaking the feet for 20 minutes before washing them.

b. Walking barefoot only on carpeted floors.

c. Applying lotion between the toes to avoid cracking of the skin.

d. Avoiding exposure of the legs and feet to sun.

ANSWERS

1. **Correct answer is c.** The National Heart, Lung and Blood Institute recommends a cholesterol level below 200 mg/dl for all adults.

a and b. These levels would be desirable but are unrealistic for most elderly people. Cholesterol levels normally increase until they peak at age 60 for men and age 70 for women. Setting unrealistic goals leads to frustration and may result in giving up on efforts to decrease cholesterol.

d. A level of 240 mg/dl reflects high cholesterol. Values between 200 mg/dl and 240 mg/dl are considered borderline high cholesterol and do not reflect a desirable goal.

2. **Correct answer is b.** A drop in BP greater than 20 mm Hg when the client stands reflects postural hypotension and puts the client at risk for falls or fainting. It requires intervention.

a. The sinoatrial (SA) node of the heart becomes less efficient with age; pulse rates in the 50's at rest are not unusual in the elderly.

c. Three consecutive readings are recommended to detect hypertension. However, the BP must be greater than 160/95 to be considered hypertension in the elderly.

d. It often takes several hours for stress-induced tachycardia to resolve in elderly clients.

3. **Correct answer is d.** The contraction of large muscles constricts veins, promoting blood flow, decreasing cardiac workload, and reducing venous pooling of blood.

a and b. Isometric exercises and weight lifting cause rapid shifts in heart rate and blood pressure that can be dangerous for the elderly.

c. Frequent position changes assist in preventing pooling of respiratory secretions and relieving pressure on skin areas but do not have cardiovascular benefits.

4. **Correct answer is c.** High alcohol intake contributes to increases in blood pressure. Hypertensive clients are usually advised to limit alcohol intake to the equivalent of 2 glasses of wine or less per day.

a. Dietary sodium should be limited in hypertensive clients. Calcium in the diet is not a contributing factor in hypertension.

b. Aerobic exercise is helpful in controlling high blood pressure. It may also contribute to weight reduction, which can help decrease blood pressure.

d. Restriction of fluid intake would be a medical order and is not appropriate advice for a nurse to give. Fluid restriction is avoided unless other measures are not successful.

5. **Correct answer is a.** Disorientation and confusion are often the first signs of digitalis toxicity in the elderly.

b and **d.** Weight gain and dyspnea are not signs of digitalis toxicity. They might indicate exacerbation of CHF.

c. Diarrhea, not constipation, is a sign of digitalis toxicity. Constipation might occur due to activity restrictions.

6. **Correct answer is d.** Dyspnea and impaired oxygenation of tissues reduce the client's ability to tolerate any amount of exercise.

a. Fluid volume excess, manifested by edema, is a more likely consequence of CHF than is fluid volume deficit.

b. Impaired verbal communication would describe dysphasia, which occurs with CVA (stroke), not CHF.

c. Acute pain may occur with CHF when exacerbations occur. Chronic pain is not a common feature of CHF.

7. **Correct answer is c.** Exercise that is within a client's tolerance should not produce angina, shortness of breath, or tachycardia.

a. Leg pain is an evaluative criterion for clients with peripheral vascular disorders, not cardiac disorders.

b and **d.** Exercise usually increases the blood pressure. A drop in blood pressure or cyanosis would signal a serious complication and would be an indication to stop exercising, but it would not be included in criteria for evaluating tolerance, since exercise should not progress quickly enough to induce such complications.

8. **Correct answer is b.** The client who has had a CVA must avoid increases in intracranial pressure, such as occur with straining at stool. Increased dietary fiber helps prevent constipation, decreasing the need for straining.

a. Intake of potassium does not affect the pathophysiology of stroke. However, diuretics, which reduce serum potassium, may be prescribed for clients with any type of cardiovascular disorder, in which case increased dietary potassium would be needed.

c. The client who has had a CVA is likely to be taking oral anticoagulants. Vitamin K would antagonize these medications and should not be increased.

d. Protein has no beneficial effect on CVA clients. Increased protein intake may increase total calorie intake, resulting in weight gain. Increased weight would add to the mobility problems if the client has hemiplegia.

9. **Correct answer is c.** Severe pain while walking describes intermittent claudication, which is the most common symptom of arteriosclerosis obliterans.

a. Rest pain would develop in the late stages of the disease.

b. Pain is much more likely than numbness with exercise. Paresthesias (including numbness) do occur, but they are more likely at rest.

d. The legs and feet of the client with arteriosclerosis obliterans become cool and pale when elevated.

10. **Correct answer is a.** Compression bandages or stockings help prevent edema and promote adequate venous blood flow and are a major element in the treatment of venous thromboembolism.

b and **c.** Bed rest is appropriate in the acute stage of venous thromboembolism. Any form of exercise to the legs would increase the risk of pulmonary emboli.

d. Heat is appropriate in the treatment of venous thromboembolism. Ice would cause vasoconstriction, worsening blood flow to the extremities.

11. **Correct answer is d.** The feet are elevated until they blanch, then dangled until they redden, then stretched out while the client is lying flat. This promotes arterial circulation to the feet.

   a. These exercises help maintain full range of motion of the ankles but are not Buerger-Allen exercises.
   b. The client with a peripheral vascular disorder should never massage the legs because of the high risk of dislodging a thrombus.
   c. While this might promote venous circulation, it does not describe Buerger-Allen exercises.

12. **Correct answer is d.** Sunburn would damage the already fragile skin, increasing the risk of ulceration and infection.

   a. Feet should not be soaked. Soaking leads to maceration, predisposing to skin breakdown or infection.
   b. The client with a peripheral vascular disorder should never walk barefoot. Small sharp objects such as pins may not be visible in carpet and could be stepped on.
   c. Lotion may be applied to dry areas of the legs and feet but must be avoided between the toes, where the excess moisture causes maceration. Ingredients in lotion provide a nutrient source for bacteria and fungi, increasing the infection risk if cracks in the skin occur.

7

Respiratory Disorders

NURSING HIGHLIGHTS

1. Normal age-related changes in the respiratory system can impair ventilation, so the nurse must plan for these potential nursing problems.
2. Incidence of upper respiratory infections and of chronic obstructive pulmonary disease (COPD) increases with age.
3. The nurse should be especially attentive to any change in respiratory status in the elderly because symptoms of respiratory diseases, such as tuberculosis and early stages of emphysema, may be absent or may be mistaken for normal age-related changes.

GLOSSARY

fremitus—a vibration that is perceptible during palpation of the lungs
pneumothorax—air or gas in the pleural cavity
tubercle—a small, rounded mass produced during *Mycobacterium* infection

I. **Age-related changes** (same as section II,B of Chapter 2)

II. **General nursing assessment**

A. General observation

See text pages

1. Check for musculoskeletal changes: Abnormal spinal curvatures may lead to diminished respiratory effectiveness. A significant increase in anteroposterior chest diameter may signal the presence of pulmonary disease.
2. Note the coloring of the client's face, neck, limbs, and nails.
    a) Ruddy complexions may be associated with chronic obstructive pulmonary disease (COPD).
    b) A blue or grayish tinge may indicate the presence of chronic bronchitis.
3. Note the client's breathing pattern, including rate, depth, rhythm, and rate of respirations while sitting, walking, changing position, and coughing.
4. Observe the client's chest during respiration to make sure that it expands symmetrically.

B. Interview

1. Inquire whether the client ever becomes short of breath while sitting quietly, walking, climbing stairs, or doing strenuous household chores.
2. Ask how many colds or other respiratory infections the client normally has in the course of a year.
3. Inquire about any breathing problems that seem to be associated with cold, heat, or dampness.
4. Ask whether the client coughs during the day and to describe the color and consistency of any mucus, phlegm, or sputum that is brought up.
5. Determine whether the client has ever smoked cigarettes (how long, brand, number per day); ask about exposure to secondhand smoke.
6. Ascertain whether the client is or has been exposed to any other form of air pollution, such as industrial chemicals, coal or asbestos dust, or excessive automobile exhaust.
7. Ask how often the client uses over-the-counter cough or cold remedies.
8. Inquire about previous immunizations for influenza and pneumonia.

C. Physical examination

1. Palpate the posterior chest to determine the depth of the client's respirations, extent of chest movement, and presence of pain or masses.
2. Check for tactile fremitus in the upper and lower lobes of the lungs.
    a) An absence of fremitus in the upper lobes may indicate pneumothorax or chronic obstructive pulmonary disease (COPD).
    b) Fremitus in the lower lobes may be a sign of masses or pneumonia.
3. Auscultate the lungs, listening for wheezes, rhonchi, and crackles.

See text pages
_____

III. Common disorders

A. Pneumonia

    1. Definition: inflammation of the lungs that is accompanied by exudation and consolidation

    2. Pathophysiology and etiology

       a) Pathophysiology: multiplication of microorganisms in the pulmonary tissue, followed by the formation of edematous fluid and other inflammatory changes; filling of the alveoli with fluid, encouraging the spread of the infection to other parts of the lungs; initially enhanced blood flow followed by diminished capillary blood flow to affected regions; gradual stiffening of the lungs, leading to atelectasis, or alveolar collapse

       b) Etiology: infection by viruses, bacteria, rickettsiae, fungi, or mycoplasmas; poor chest expansion; shallow breathing; other respiratory diseases that cause bronchial obstruction and mucus formation; aspiration of foreign material

    3. Symptoms: restlessness; confusion; changes in behavior; pleuritic pain, which may be absent or slight in the elderly client; temperature elevation, which may be absent or late in the elderly client; cough; increased respiratory rate; tachycardia; fatigue

    4. Treatment: preventive care, including annual vaccination against influenza viruses and one-time pneumococcal vaccination for those over 65; antibiotics; supportive care, including bed rest and administration of abundant (but not excessive) fluids and analgesics; supplementary oxygenation; monitoring for complications (e.g., congestive heart failure, paralytic ileus, empyema, pleurisy, hypotension, hypoxia, shock, septicemia); endotracheal intubation or tracheotomy (in severe cases)

B. Chronic obstructive pulmonary disease (COPD)

    1. Chronic bronchitis

       a) Definition

          (1) Recurrent inflammation of the bronchi due to repeated attacks of acute bronchitis or to chronic disease

          (2) Characterized by coughing, expectoration, and changes in lung tissue

       b) Pathophysiology and etiology

          (1) Pathophysiology: increased edema, secretions, and bronchospasm; impaired mucociliary clearance; diffuse airway obstruction due to thickening of bronchial walls

          (2) Etiology: smoking; history of bronchial asthma, pneumonia, or influenza; exposure to industrial pollutants

       c) Symptoms: persistent cough, expectoration of thick white mucus, shortness of breath (increased by cold or dampness), frequent acute respiratory infections, sensation of heaviness in the chest, expectoration of sputum that may be streaked with blood (in advanced cases), hypoxia, emphysema

  d) Treatment: prevention of further irritation of the bronchial mucosa; immunization against influenza; elimination of smoking; avoidance of industrial pollutants; increased fluid intake; eating of balanced diet; administration of bronchodilators, antibiotics, and/or steroids; postural drainage; chest percussion

2. Emphysema
  a) Definition: a chronic disease marked by progressive destruction of the walls of the alveoli; diagnosed in the elderly when there is an obstructive pattern during forced expiration
  b) Pathophysiology and etiology
    (1) Pathophysiology: gradual decrease in the number of alveoli and in the surface area of the pulmonary membrane, leading to abnormally enlarged air spaces and limited airflow from the lungs; inflammation and swelling of bronchi
    (2) Etiology: chronic bronchitis, cigarette smoking, sustained exposure to air pollutants, familial predisposition (in some clients)
  c) Symptoms: dyspnea not relieved by sitting, chronic cough, fatigue, weakness, distention of neck veins during expiration, anorexia, weight loss

---

✔ CLIENT TEACHING CHECKLIST ✔

Emphysema Management for the Elderly Client

Because they often must make drastic modifications to lifelong habits, elderly clients with emphysema require extensive emotional support and teaching. Discuss the following guidelines with older clients who have emphysema:

✔ If you smoke, stop now. Participating in a smoking-cessation class may be helpful.
✔ Eat a well-balanced diet and drink plenty of fluids.
✔ Practice all the breathing exercises that have been prescribed.
✔ Take all prescribed medications, even when you are feeling well.
✔ Do not overuse bronchodilators that are prescribed to be taken as needed; excessive use (3–4 times a day) has been linked to increased incidence of death and morbidity.
✔ Try to avoid stressful situations.
✔ Alternate periods of activity and rest.
✔ Stay indoors when it is extremely cold and avoid drafts.
✔ Immediately report any sign of respiratory infection, however minor, to your physician (e.g., a change in the color or character of sputum).
✔ Do not take over-the-counter sleeping aids or other medications without your doctor's permission.

      d) Treatment: smoking cessation; prevention of and immediate medical attention for respiratory infections; positive-pressure breathing exercises; postural drainage; administration of bronchodilators; low-flow oxygen therapy; supportive care, including a well-balanced diet and adequate fluid intake (see Client Teaching Checklist, "Emphysema Management for the Elderly Client"); administration of corticosteroids (in severe cases)

  C. Tuberculosis (TB)
    1. Definition: a highly communicable infectious disease characterized by the formation of tubercles and necrosis of tissue
    2. Pathophysiology and etiology
      a) Pathophysiology: exudation in response to multiplication of the tubercle bacillus in the alveoli or bronchi; surrounding of inflamed areas with collagen, lymphocytes, and fibroblasts; progression of necrosis within the infected area; liquefaction or calcification of necrotic tissue
      b) Etiology: infection with *Mycobacterium tuberculosis,* reactivation of previous infection
    3. Symptoms
      a) Early stage: fatigue; anorexia; weakness; weight loss; slight, nonproductive cough
      b) Later stages: elevated temperature and night sweats, which may be absent in the elderly; cough that produces blood-streaked sputum and purulent mucus; wasting; dyspnea; chest pain
    4. Treatment: sustained therapy with multiple antituberculous drugs (see Client Teaching Checklist, "Adverse Effects of Antituberculous Drugs"); supportive care, including well-balanced diet and adequate rest; surgical treatment, including segmental resection, wedge resection, lobectomy, or pneumonectomy

IV. Essential nursing care

See text pages
_____

A. Nursing assessment (see section II of this chapter)

B. Nursing diagnoses
    1. Ineffective airway clearance related to obstruction or inelasticity of lungs
    2. Fluid volume deficit related to fever and diaphoresis
    3. Altered nutrition, less than body requirements, related to anorexia
    4. Impaired physical mobility related to fatigue or dyspnea
    5. High risk for infection related to chronic respiratory disease
    6. Anxiety related to breathing problems
    7. Noncompliance with antituberculous drug therapy

C. Nursing implementation (intervention)
 1. Encourage the client to preserve remaining respiratory capacity by following prescribed treatment regimen, including medication and abdominal and pursed-lip breathing exercises (see Client Teaching Checklist, "Deep-Breathing Exercises," in Chapter 1).
 2. Discuss the importance of increased fluid intake with the client; for a hospitalized or institutionalized client, offer fluids frequently, measure intake and output, and notify the physician if urinary output is less than 30 ml/hour.
 3. Encourage the client who smokes to attend smoking-cessation classes.
 4. Supplement the meals of clients who habitually eat poorly with high-protein, high-calorie formulations; if necessary, provide calories and electrolytes as ordered with short-term intravenous solutions.
 5. Assist the client with limited mobility in scheduling daily tasks around rest periods; help identify family members or outside resources to help with shopping, home maintenance, and other strenuous tasks.
 6. Teach the client who is limited to chair or bed rest the importance of coughing and deep-breathing exercises.
 7. Teach the client to avoid infection by eating a well-balanced diet, getting adequate rest, avoiding temperature extremes, and limiting contact with family members or friends who have respiratory infections and to recognize the earliest signs of respiratory infection.
 8. When noncompliance with drug therapy is known or suspected, attempt to determine the reasons for the client's behavior, and help the client devise a system for remembering to take medications as ordered (e.g., recording when each dose is taken).

✔ CLIENT TEACHING CHECKLIST ✔

Adverse Effects of Antituberculous Drugs

Explain to the elderly client that the following adverse effects of antituberculous drugs should be reported to the physician at once:

Isoniazid
✔ Gastrointestinal distress
✔ Peripheral neuropathy
✔ Hyperglycemia

Para-aminosalicylic acid
✔ Gastrointestinal irritation
✔ Anorexia
✔ Nausea
✔ Vomiting
✔ Diarrhea

Rifampin
✔ Gastrointestinal distress
✔ Headache

✔ Drowsiness
✔ Ataxia
✔ Dizziness
✔ Confusion
✔ Visual disturbances
✔ Muscular weakness
✔ Fever
✔ Urticaria

Streptomycin
✔ Hearing impairment
✔ Disequilibrium (can lead to falls and other safety hazards)

D. Nursing evaluation
   1. The client's respiratory capacity increases.
   2. The client stops smoking.
   3. The client maintains adequate hydration.
   4. The client maintains adequate food intake.
   5. The client maintains daily activities to tolerance level.
   6. The client verbalizes guidelines for avoiding and recognizing respiratory infection.
   7. The client's temperature remains normal and he/she exhibits no other signs of respiratory infection.
   8. The client correctly describes and complies with drug regimen.

E. Gerontologic nursing considerations
   1. The elderly have reduced ability to fight off infection and to manage it once it occurs; they are also more susceptible to infection when under stress.
   2. Confusion, restlessness, and behavior changes are key pneumonia symptoms in the elderly because blood is diverted from the brain to fight the infection.
   3. There is normal decline of blood oxygen (PO_2) with aging, but blood carbon dioxide (PCO_2) and bicarbonate levels should remain normal.
   4. Be aware that chronic obstructive pulmonary disease (COPD) may be present in elderly clients hospitalized for other conditions and should be part of care plan.
   5. It is important to emphasize forced expiration since effective expiration is difficult for the elderly.
   6. Carefully evaluate the cause of low-grade fevers and night sweats in elderly clients; these 2 symptoms of tuberculosis (TB) may not be evident because of impaired thermoregulation and reduced diaphoresis.
   7. The 2-step tuberculin skin test, which is used to ascertain whether TB infection has existed in the body at some time, is recommended for clients over 50 due to weakened antibody reactions.
   8. Risk factors for a reactivated TB infection among the elderly include chronic disease, alcoholism, malnutrition, diabetes, cancer, and decreased resistance due to age-related decline in immune levels.
   9. Reassure fearful elderly clients who have TB that they will not have to be institutionalized as was done in the past.

1. Which of the following should be considered abnormal in the elderly client?

   a. Increased residual volume
   b. Diminished breath sounds at the bases
   c. Increased anteroposterior chest diameter
   d. A nonproductive cough

2. While examining an elderly client, the nurse observes a ruddy complexion. Based on this finding, the nurse should assess for other signs and symptoms of:

   a. Pneumonia.
   b. Chronic obstructive pulmonary disease (COPD).
   c. Tuberculosis (TB).
   d. Pneumothorax.

3. Elderly clients with pneumonia are most likely to exhibit:

   a. Severe pleuritic pain.
   b. High fever.
   c. Increasing confusion.
   d. Decreased respiratory rate.

4. Which of the following symptoms should the nurse anticipate in an elderly client diagnosed with chronic bronchitis?

   a. Nonproductive cough
   b. Shortness of breath increased by damp weather
   c. Dyspnea not relieved by sitting up
   d. Night sweats

5. Ninety-year-old Mr. Addison is weak and anorexic and has a temperature of 99.8°F. Upon admission to a nursing home, he has a questionable tuberculin test and an inconclusive chest x-ray. Tuberculosis (TB) is suspected. Because Mr. Addison is unable to cough up sputum, the nurse should anticipate that which of the following diagnostic tests may be ordered?

   a. Pulmonary function testing
   b. Arterial blood gases

   c. Gastric content analysis
   d. Bronchoscopy

6. Which of the following psychosocial responses is most commonly seen in elderly adults who have been diagnosed with tuberculosis (TB)?

   a. Social isolation related to fear of infecting others
   b. Ineffective individual coping related to excessive dependency
   c. Severe anxiety related to poor prognosis
   d. High risk for self-directed violence related to diagnosis of chronic illness

7. The elderly client being treated with streptomycin for tuberculosis (TB) should have which of the following checked periodically during therapy?

   a. Color vision
   b. Visual acuity
   c. Hearing
   d. Peripheral touch sensation

8. Which of the following would be appropriate to teach the elderly client with emphysema?

   a. Limit your fluid intake to 1.5 liters or less daily.
   b. Stay indoors and avoid drafts during cold weather.
   c. Report a cough that produces white sputum to your physician.
   d. When you inhale, your chest should rise and your abdomen should not.

9. Immunizations recommended for elderly clients whose respiratory function is compromised include which of the following?

   a. Pneumococcus
   b. *Haemophilus influenzae* B (Hib)
   c. Bacillus Calmette-Guérin (BCG)
   d. Diphtheria-pertussis-tetanus (DPT)

10. Which of the following modifications should be considered when postural drainage is prescribed for an elderly client?

   a. Cough suppressants should be administered before the procedure.

   b. Percussion and vibration are eliminated to prevent injury to fragile bones.

   c. Oxygen administration should be discontinued during the procedure.

   d. The prone position with head down should be eliminated.

11. Which of the following is an appropriate instruction regarding breathing exercises to be given to an elderly client with chronic obstructive pulmonary disease (COPD)?

   a. Hold your abdomen still while your chest rises.

   b. Inhale through your mouth rather than your nose.

   c. Inhale before an activity and exhale during the activity.

   d. Inhalation should last twice as long as exhalation.

12. When evaluating the client's use of a PRN aerosol nebulizer (metered-dose inhaler), which of the following would indicate a need for additional teaching?

   a. The client places the inhaler in a bowl of water to determine whether it is empty.

   b. The client seals the lips around the mouthpiece when inhaling the medication.

   c. The client limits use of the inhaler to no more than twice daily.

   d. The client uses both hands to squeeze the inhaler to release the medication.

ANSWERS

1. **Correct answer is d.** Any cough is abnormal for a client of any age. A cough should always be investigated.

   a. Increased residual volume is a normal age-related change brought about by decreased muscle strength of the thorax.

   b. Incomplete lung expansion is a normal age-related change and often results in collapse of the bases, which is reflected in diminished breath sounds at the bases.

   c. Some increase in anteroposterior chest diameter is common with aging, especially as kyphosis develops. A large increase may reflect chronic obstructive pulmonary disease (COPD).

2. **Correct answer is b.** Ruddy complexion is often associated with COPD, especially emphysema, in which hypoxia and increased carbon dioxide (CO_2) levels occur.

   a and d. The client with pneumonia or pneumothorax is more likely to exhibit pallor or cyanosis associated with impaired oxygenation.

   c. Color changes are not usually associated with TB, since oxygenation is not severely impaired until late in the disease process.

3. **Correct answer is c.** Increasing confusion reflects decreased cerebral oxygenation. Because the elderly do not have as much respiratory reserve capacity as younger clients, any disease process is likely to result in inadequate oxygenation.

   a. Pain is often slight in the elderly and may be ignored or treated by the client as normal for his/her age.

   b. Altered thermoregulation and a normally lower body temperature in the elderly result in less significant temperature elevations in response to infection than in younger clients.

   d. Increased respiratory rate is a common symptom of pneumonia in the elderly.

4. **Correct answer is b.** In the client with chronic bronchitis, shortness of breath is typically increased by exposure to cold or damp weather.

   a. The cough in chronic bronchitis is usually productive of thick white sputum.

   c. Dyspnea that is not relieved when sitting up is typical of emphysema.

   d. Night sweats are typical of tuberculosis (TB).

5. **Correct answer is c.** Because Mr. Addison has a weak cough that does not raise sputum into the mouth to be expectorated, the sputum test cannot be done. However, as the sputum of a client in this condition is often swallowed, analysis of the gastric contents will reveal the presence of TB organisms, despite the apparently nonproductive cough.

   a and b. Neither arterial blood gases nor pulmonary function tests would produce conclusive information for diagnosis of TB.
   d. Bronchoscopy is an invasive procedure and would not be used for an elderly client if other less invasive diagnostic methods are available.

6. **Correct answer is a.** The elderly were raised in an era when TB-infected individuals were sent to sanatoriums to segregate them from others, since adequate antimicrobial treatments were not available. They may not understand that adequate treatment eliminates the risk of infecting others and may voluntarily avoid contact with family and friends.

   b. There is no reason to expect that an individual receiving proper treatment would be more dependent than usual. The elderly are more likely to attempt to maintain their independence.
   c. The prognosis is excellent when TB is diagnosed and treated appropriately.
   d. TB is not a chronic disease; with treatment it can be cured. There has been no indication of increased suicide rates in the elderly with TB.

7. **Correct answer is c.** Streptomycin is an aminoglycoside and may damage the inner ear. Hearing impairment may also alert the nurse to assess for vertigo or gait problems resulting from damage to the vestibular system.

   a. Testing color vision would be appropriate for ethambutol.
   b. Visual acuity is not affected by antitubercular drugs.

   d. Testing peripheral touch sensation would be appropriate for isoniazid (INH), which causes peripheral neuropathy.

8. **Correct answer is b.** The shortness of breath with emphysema is exacerbated by exposure to cold. A drafty environment increases the risk of upper respiratory infections.

   a. Fluid intake should be increased to help thin and mobilize respiratory secretions.
   c. White or clear sputum is normally produced by clients with chronic obstructive pulmonary disease (COPD). If the sputum color changes, it should be reported, as it may signal infection.
   d. Diaphragmatic breathing, in which the abdomen rises with inhalation, is appropriate for a client with emphysema.

9. **Correct answer is a.** Pneumococcus pneumonia is a relatively common problem in the elderly and can be prevented with appropriate immunization.

   b. Hib is a childhood immunization recommended to protect infants against the meningitis caused by the *Haemophilus influenzae* organism. Polyvalent influenza virus vaccine is recommended for the elderly.
   c. BCG is recommended in countries where TB is endemic. Although the incidence is increasing in the United States, the vaccine is not recommended for everyone, since it makes the usual screening tests invalid.
   d. DT (diphtheria-tetanus) should be administered every 10 years to all adults. Pertussis vaccine (included in DPT) is indicated only in childhood.

10. **Correct answer is d.** For many elderly clients, lying prone or with the head down is stressful and may increase oxygen demand. Arthritic changes may prevent the use of this position. Some neurologic and cardiovascular disorders contraindicate this position.

    a. Cough suppressants should not be used before the treatment. Postural drainage is intended to mobilize secretions so they can be coughed up and expectorated.

b. Percussion and vibration help mobilize secretions. They need to be done gently for the elderly client but are not contraindicated.

c. The elderly person who becomes dyspneic with activity needs oxygen administered during the procedure to prevent hypoxia.

11. **Correct answer is c.** Inhaling before and exhaling during activity helps prevent holding one's breath, which is contraindicated.

   a. Diaphragmatic breathing is prescribed for clients with COPD. The chest should remain still while the abdomen rises.

   b. The client should close the mouth and inhale through the nose.

   d. Exhalation should last twice as long as inhalation since the elderly frequently do not exhale efficiently.

12. **Correct answer is b.** This method results in deposition of much of the medication in the mouth. The lips should be partly open to allow air to be drawn in with the medication. The air carries the medication into the bronchial passages. For the elderly, whose respiratory effort is not as strong as that of younger people, this is especially important.

   a. This is the correct way to determine how much medication remains in the inhaler because an empty inhaler floats.

   c. Excessive use of PRN bronchodilators, even 3–4 times a day, has been associated with an increase in serious adverse effects in the elderly.

   d. Because the elderly often have weakened grip strength, use of both hands may be necessary to provide a strong enough squeezing action to release medication.

8

Gastrointestinal and Genitourinary Disorders

NURSING HIGHLIGHTS

1. Because older people may accept gastrointestinal problems as a normal part of aging, the nurse should ask carefully worded interview questions to detect disorders a client may not think to discuss.
2. Incontinence is not an inevitable result of aging; it can be successfully managed in most elderly clients.
3. The incidence of urinary tract infections increases with age. Such infections are the most common type among the elderly.
4. Because of the embarrassment the elderly may experience related to urologic and gynecologic issues such as incontinence and sexual dysfunction, they often may not be reported. The nurse should be sensitive and patient in questioning elderly clients about these issues.

GLOSSARY

costovertebral angle—the junction of the lower portion of the rib cage and vertebral column
diverticulum (pl. diverticula)—protrusion or pouch in the colon, stomach, esophagus, or small intestine
osteomalacia—condition causing softening of the bone
stria (pl. striae)—pink, purplish, or white line of atrophic tissue on the breasts, thighs, abdomen, and buttocks, caused by the weakening of elastic dermal tissues; associated with obesity, tumors, Cushing's disease, and long-term use of corticosteroids

ENHANCED OUTLINE

See text pages
_____

I. Gastrointestinal (GI) disorders

A. Age-related changes (see section II,C of Chapter 2)

B. General nursing assessment
  1. General observation
     a) Observe the client's general appearance and bearing, noting signs of fatigue or weakness, which can indicate the presence of internal bleeding, malnutrition, or fluid and electrolyte imbalance.
     b) Observe the client for unusual thinness or obesity, which may signal poor dietary habits.
     c) Note the client's coloring; pallor may be a sign of GI bleeding.
     d) Note the condition of the client's skin.
        (1) Discoloration, scaling, rashes, or signs of scratching may indicate nutritional deficiencies.
        (2) Dry skin with poor turgor may be a sign of malnutrition or dehydration.
     e) Be attentive for halitosis, which is associated with poor oral hygiene, oral and esophageal disease, lung infection or abscess, uremia, and liver disorders.
  2. Interview
     a) Inquire about the client's dental hygiene, including means of caring for teeth or dentures, frequency of visits to the dentist, and any bleeding, hypersensitivity, or pain.
     b) Ask the client to describe his/her typical daily food intake, known food allergies, any intolerance to specific foods, and any changes in the taste of foods, appetite, or weight.
     c) Inquire about instances of indigestion, what provokes it, and how the client controls it (e.g., use of digestive aids).
     d) Ask about bowel habits, the color and consistency of stools, the presence of blood, the need to strain, and frequency of use of laxatives or enemas.
     e) Determine whether the client experiences any of the common signs of GI disease (e.g., sore mouth, difficulty in swallowing, burning in the stomach or intestines, nausea, vomiting, diarrhea, constipation).
  3. Physical examination
     a) Check the color, moisture, and general condition of the lips, especially noting bluish discoloration and fissures and cracks.

b) Inspect the mouth for dryness; irritation; swollen, bleeding gums; ill-fitting dentures; and broken or decayed teeth.

c) Check the tongue for any deviation or atrophy, unusual smoothness or redness, any coating, and thick white patches or other lesions.

d) Evaluate the client's swallowing reflex by pressing a tongue depressor on the middle of the tongue, asking the client to say "ah," and noting whether the soft palate rises to block the nasopharynx and whether the uvula stays midline.

e) Ask the client to lie supine and examine the abdomen for rashes, indentations, striae, and asymmetrical distention.

f) Listen for bowel sounds and palpate the abdomen to detect the presence of masses.

g) Examine the rectum for signs of poor hygiene, inflammation, hemorrhoids, fissures, tumors, or fecal impaction.

h) Obtain a stool sample. Check color, consistency, and presence of blood or mucus.

C. Common disorders
  1. Malnutrition
    a) Definition: poor nourishment resulting from inadequate, excessive, or imbalanced dietary intake or from a metabolic disorder
    b) Pathophysiology and etiology
      (1) Pathophysiology: persistent negative nitrogen balance associated with continuous conversion of protein to glucose, leading to steady loss of muscle tissue
      (2) Etiology: see Chapter 1, section VI,A; also, slower peristalsis, reduced secretion of gastric acid, decreased absorption of nutrients (e.g., iron, vitamin B_{12}, calcium) due to reduced intestinal blood flow and decreased cells in the intestinal absorbing surface
    c) Symptoms: weight loss of more than 5% during previous month or 10% in previous 6 months, weight that is 10% below or 20% above ideal range, serum albumin level lower than 3.5 g/100 ml, hemoglobin level below 12 g/dl, hematocrit value below 35%, fatigue, lethargy, hair loss, dermatitis
    d) Treatment: monitoring of weight, food intake, and laboratory values; client education and counseling about good nutrition; administration of appropriate vitamin and mineral supplements; treatment of malnutrition-related medical and dental problems (e.g., obstructive disorder, ill-fitting dentures)
  2. Lactose intolerance
    a) Definition: malabsorption of the lactose (milk sugar) in milk and possibly in other dairy products
    b) Pathophysiology and etiology
      (1) Pathophysiology: inability to digest lactose due to insufficiency of the enzyme lactase

        (2) Etiology: genetic predisposition, age-related deficiency in lactose production

  c) Symptoms: flatulence, bloating, intestinal cramping, and/or diarrhea after ingestion of ≥8 oz milk or other dairy product

  d) Treatment: elimination of milk/dairy products, inclusion of dietary sources of calcium (e.g., greens, dried beans), administration of lactase before ingestion of dairy products

3. Dental problems

  a) Definition: disease of the teeth, gums, or other tissues within the oral cavity that affects eating and speaking

  b) Pathophysiology and etiology

    (1) Pathophysiology: breakdown of tooth enamel, absorption of dental roots, tooth malocclusion, gum atrophy or hyperplasia, poor mastication, neoplastic growths

    (2) Etiology: excessive intake of sweets, vitamin B deficiency, diabetes, osteomalacia, hormonal disorders, hyperparathyroidism, Cushing's disease

  c) Symptoms: oral pain or sensitivity, halitosis, decreased food intake, malnutrition, constipation, systemic infection

  d) Treatment: dental care, oral hygiene instruction, treatment of underlying disease (e.g., infection, diabetes)

4. Dysphagia

  a) Definition: difficulty swallowing, with increased risk of aspiration

  b) Pathophysiology and etiology

    (1) Pathophysiology: structural or functional changes in the mouth, pharynx, or esophagus that alter swallowing dynamics

    (2) Etiology: stroke-related hemiplegia or muscular weakness, dementia (late stages), Parkinson's and other neuromuscular diseases, spastic tongue associated with medication-induced tardive dyskinesia, chronic lung disease (late stages)

  c) Symptoms: drooling or leaking of food from mouth, pouching of food in cheeks, nasal regurgitation, signs of aspiration after swallowing (e.g., red face, teary eyes, cough), complaint of lump in throat

  d) Treatment: use of thickened fluids; use of therapeutic feeding techniques

5. Hiatal hernia

  a) Definition: protrusion of part of the stomach above the diaphragm

  b) Pathophysiology and etiology

    (1) Pathophysiology: rolling or sliding of a portion of the stomach through a weakened portion of the diaphragm

      (2) Etiology: congenital diaphragm weakness, trauma, obesity, multiple pregnancies; prevalent among women over 60

  c) Symptoms: *may be asymptomatic in the elderly;* when seen, dysphagia; belching; heartburn; regurgitation; aspiration; vomiting; substernal or epigastric pressure after eating, especially when lying down; bleeding; substernal pain; iron deficiency anemia

  d) Treatment: weight reduction; bland diet; small, frequent meals; administration of antacids, cimetidine (Tagamet), famotidine (Pepcid), and ranitidine hydrochloride (Zantac); treatment of iron deficiency anemia; surgery (rare)

6. Diverticular disease
  a) Definition
    (1) Diverticulosis: existence of multiple pouches or herniations in the wall of the colon
    (2) Diverticulitis: inflammation or infection of diverticula
  b) Pathophysiology and etiology
    (1) Pathophysiology
      (a) Diverticulosis: gradual response to high pressures generated in the sigmoid colon
      (b) Diverticulitis: trapping of undigested food or bacteria in the diverticula, leading to diminished blood supply, infection, perforation, and formation of a local abscess; intra-abdominal perforation and peritonitis in severe cases
    (2) Etiology
      (a) Diverticulosis: chronic constipation, obesity, hiatal hernia, age-related atrophy of intestinal wall muscles
      (b) Diverticulitis: overeating, straining at stool, consumption of irritating foods and alcohol; common in older men
  c) Symptoms
    (1) Diverticulosis: *often asymptomatic;* occasional bleeding
    (2) Diverticulitis: pain in the left lower quadrant, nausea, vomiting, diarrhea, low-grade fever, blood or mucus in the stool
  d) Treatment
    (1) Diverticulosis: bland diet, adequate hydration, weight reduction, avoidance of constipation
    (2) Diverticulitis: in acute or active phase, control of infection, adequate nutrition (through clear liquids or nasogastric tube and/or intravenous fluids), pain relief, rest, bowel resection or temporary colostomy (in severe cases); in maintenance phase, low-residue diet until symptoms disappear, then selected high-fiber diet (no nuts, seeds, corn, tomatoes)

7. Chronic constipation
  a) Definition: repeatedly difficult or infrequent evacuation of feces
  b) Pathophysiology and etiology
    (1) Pathophysiology: delayed transit of feces through the large intestine
    (2) Etiology (see Chapter 1, section VIII,A,2,a)

        c) Symptoms: passage of hard, dry, infrequent stools; difficult elimination; diarrhea

        d) Treatment: promotion of dietary habits that encourage normal defecation, adequate fluid intake, sufficient exercise, provision of adequate time for elimination on a set schedule, use of a stool chart, short-term use of laxatives and enemas, treatment of underlying disorder

    8. Colon cancer

        a) Definition: neoplastic growth in the large intestine, most often found in the sigmoid colon and rectum; incidence increases with age

        b) Pathophysiology and etiology

            (1) Pathophysiology: gradual development from an adenomatous polyp, followed by spread into the layers of the bowel wall, enlargement into the bowel lumen, or circulation through the lymphatics or blood

            (2) Etiology: diet that is high in fat and refined carbohydrates and low in fiber, family history of polyposis or chronic ulcerative colitis

        c) Symptoms: change in bowel function, bloody stools, epigastric pain, nausea, anorexia, jaundice, presence of mass upon digital rectal examination

        d) Treatment: colostomy, resection with anastomosis, radiation therapy, chemotherapy with fluorouracil and leucovorin calcium

  D. Essential nursing care

    1. Nursing assessment (see section I,B of this chapter)

    2. Nursing diagnoses

        a) Altered nutrition, less than body requirements, related to altered taste sensations

        b) Altered nutrition, more than body requirements, related to lack of income to purchase healthful foods

        c) Activity intolerance related to vitamin and mineral deficiencies

        d) High risk for aspiration related to dysphagia

        e) Fluid volume deficit related to infection

        f) Constipation related to improper diet or poor hydration

        g) Pain related to intestinal obstruction

        h) Anxiety related to colostomy procedure

    3. Nursing implementation (intervention)

        a) See section VI,B of Chapter 1 for nursing interventions to prevent or treat poor nutritional habits.

        b) Provide instruction in proper oral hygiene.

    c) For the client with dysphagia, instruct the client to tip the head forward (chin to chest) while swallowing and to always eat sitting up.

    d) For the client with hiatal hernia, instruct the client not to lie down for 1–2 hours after a meal, not to have a bedtime snack, to avoid constricting clothing (e.g., girdle), and to sleep without pillows and with head of bed elevated on blocks.

    e) Monitor fluid and electrolyte balance.

    f) See section VIII,B,2,a-b of Chapter 1 for interventions to prevent or treat constipation.

    g) Assist the client with physical and psychologic adjustment to colostomy procedure. Refer the client to a support group.

    h) For any gastrointestinal (GI) disorder, instruct the client about proper diet and proper methods of taking medications; provide client education about common drug side effects.

4. Nursing evaluation

    a) The client consumes balanced meals that are appropriate for body size and activity level.

    b) The client performs activities of daily living (ADLs) to tolerance.

    c) The client maintains normal hydration.

    d) The client eliminates stool of consistent amount and texture, on a predictable schedule, without discomfort or straining.

    e) The client states that pain is reduced.

    f) The client states that anxiety regarding colostomy has been alleviated.

5. Gerontologic nursing considerations

    a) Explain to older clients that they can often avoid GI problems by eating 5–6 small meals per day rather than the traditional 3 meals and by scheduling their main meal at midday.

    b) Elderly clients are more susceptible than younger adults to adverse effects from the use of cimetidine (see Nurse Alert, "Side Effects of Cimetidine in Elderly Clients").

      c) In elderly clients who are receiving gastric feedings over a prolonged period, be alert to the presence of complications related to gastric tube use (e.g., ulceration, respiratory infection). Continually monitor for the need to continue nasogastric or intravenous feeding method.

      d) Dependence on laxatives, which can cause dehydration and electrolyte loss, is a problem for the elderly because many older clients mistakenly assume that daily evacuation is necessary for good health. The nurse should explain that the range of normal varies by individual.

      e) Because many GI problems among the elderly are related to insufficient funds, help the client in need to obtain services (e.g., low-cost dental care, transportation to medical and dental appointments, nutrition or meal programs).

See text pages

_____

II. Genitourinary disorders

A. Age-related changes (see section II,E of Chapter 2)

B. General nursing assessment
1. General observation: With the client in a sitting and a supine position, inspect the abdomen and costovertebral angle, noting any asymmetry or discoloration.
2. Interview
    a) Determine the client's urination pattern.
    b) Ask the client about color, clarity, and odor of his/her urine.
    c) Inquire whether the client ever loses control of his/her urine or if the bladder fails to empty fully after voiding.
    d) Determine whether the client has felt pain, burning, or itching in the lower abdomen or genital area.
    e) Ask if the client experiences discharge from the genitals.
    f) In female clients, determine history of pregnancies, menopause, lumps, cancer, and sexually transmitted diseases (STDs) and dates of last breast self-exam, Pap smear, and mammogram.
    g) In male clients, determine history of prostate problems and STDs.
    h) Inquire about the client's sexual function.
3. Physical examination
    a) Palpate and percuss the abdomen for bladder fullness, pelvic discomfort, or other abnormalities.
    b) Inspect the genitals for inflammation or edema.
    c) Inspect the scrotum for symmetry.
    d) Inspect the vagina for excessive discharge, bleeding, color, or odor.

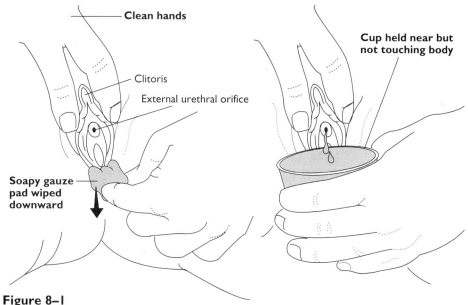

Clean hands

Clitoris

External urethral orifice

Cup held near but not touching body

Soapy gauze pad wiped downward

Figure 8–1
Method for Collecting Clean-Catch Urine Sample

e) Palpate the genitals for lesions or masses.
f) Palpate the breasts or prostate for masses.
g) Collect a clean-catch midstream urine specimen; catheterize if necessary to get sample.

C. Common disorders
  1. Urinary disorders
    a) Definition: reduced control of urination, including incontinence, urgency, and frequency
    b) Pathophysiology and etiology
      (1) Pathophysiology: replacement of smooth muscle and elastic tissue in bladder with fibrous connective tissue, decreased bladder capacity, bladder neck obstructions, decreased sphincter tone
      (2) Etiology: age-related changes, neurologic disorders, urinary infection, dementia, sedation, pelvic or bladder tumors, enlargement of prostate, diverticulitis (see also Chapter 1, section VIII,A,1)
    c) Symptoms: involuntary loss of urine, sudden need to urinate, need to urinate frequently
    d) Treatment: management of underlying medical problem(s), scheduled toileting, improvement of mobility, Kegel exercises (see Client Teaching Checklist, "Kegel Exercises"), Credé's maneuver, biofeedback, drug therapy (e.g., anticholinergics, adrenergic antagonists), surgical interventions

2. Urinary tract infection (UTI)
    a) Definition: inflammation of 1 or more urinary tract structures
    b) Pathophysiology and etiology
        (1) Pathophysiology: decrease in strength of bladder muscles leading to incomplete bladder emptying and establishment of gram-negative bacteria in urine residue; altered antigen-antibody response leading to generalized age-related reduction of resistance to infection
        (2) Etiology: benign prostatic hypertrophy, diverticula of bladder, bladder stones, contaminated urologic instruments, fecal contamination, indwelling catheters, immobility
    c) Symptoms: urinary urgency and/or frequency; burning or pain when urinating; perineal, suprapubic, or lower back pain (pain often less severe in elderly clients than in younger adults); hematuria; chills; fever (may be late or absent in the elderly)
    d) Treatment: correction of contributing factors; antimicrobial therapy (usually with sulfonamide); removal of partial obstruction, if present
3. Vaginitis
    a) Definition: inflammation of the vagina
    b) Pathophysiology and etiology
        (1) Pathophysiology: thinning of the vaginal epithelium and loss of tissue elasticity, reduction of and rise in pH of vaginal secretions, change in intravaginal flora

---

✔ CLIENT TEACHING CHECKLIST ✔

Kegel Exercises

Explanation to the client:

✔ Alternately squeeze and relax pubococcygeal muscle (muscle that is tensed to stop urinary flow while voiding) for 3 seconds at a time.
✔ Begin with a series of 10 squeezes once a day.
✔ Increase until doing a series of 10 3–4 times a day.

Special notes:

✔ Exercises are most effective when muscles of buttocks and thighs are not used.
✔ Exercises should not be done while urinating—may cause infection.
✔ Exercises can be done lying on back with a pillow under the knees or while sitting or standing.

      (2) Etiology: age-related changes, long-term corticosteroid therapy, poorly controlled diabetes

   c) Symptoms: vaginal redness, soreness, burning, pruritus, and discharge, painful intercourse; in severe cases, bleeding and adhesions

   d) Treatment: administration of local estrogen suppositories or creams, acid douches, good hygiene

  4. Benign prostatic hypertrophy

   a) Definition: enlargement of the prostate

   b) Pathophysiology and etiology

      (1) Pathophysiology: periurethral hyperplasia that decreases diameter of prostatic urethra

      (2) Etiology: advancing age, possible hormonal imbalance

   c) Symptoms: *may be asymptomatic initially;* in presence of obstruction, urinary hesitancy, narrowed stream, straining to void, frequency, urgency, nocturia, hematuria, cystitis

   d) Treatment: administration of finasteride (Proscar), antiandrogen preparations, or progestational agents; catheterization; suprapubic cystostomy; transcystoscopic urethroplasty; complete or partial prostatectomy

D. Essential nursing care

  1. Nursing assessment (see section II,B of this chapter)

  2. Nursing diagnoses

   a) Disturbance in self-concept related to urinary incontinence

   b) Hyperthermia related to UTI

   c) Anxiety related to possible loss of sexual function

   d) Altered urinary elimination related to prostatic enlargement

   e) Sleep pattern disturbance related to nocturia or urinary retention

  3. Nursing implementation (intervention)

   a) See section VIII,B,1 of Chapter 1 for interventions for urinary incontinence.

   b) Monitor intake and output of the client with UTI; force fluids if not contraindicated by cardiac condition.

   c) Administer antibiotics as ordered to resolve UTI.

   d) Suggest daily use of cranberry juice to acidify urine.

   e) Instruct the client in hygiene practices that can help prevent UTIs and vaginitis (e.g., for females, wiping front to back).

   f) Teach the female client about proper medication application methods to treat vaginitis.

   g) Dispel possible misconceptions of the male client that benign prostatic hypertrophy is an inescapable part of the aging process and that surgical intervention is likely to cause impotence.

   h) Explain measures for minimizing nocturia and facilitating urination in the client with benign prostatic hypertrophy.

  4. Nursing evaluation

   a) The client demonstrates reduction of episodes of incontinence.

   b) The client is free from infection.

      c) The client is able to use vaginal medications correctly.

      d) The client resumes customary sexual activity.

      e) The client urinates without discomfort or difficulty.

      f) The client gets sufficient amount of uninterrupted sleep.

5. Gerontologic nursing considerations

      a) Slight abnormalities in renal function tests (e.g., unreliable proteinuria and glycosuria readings) are common in elderly clients and must be accounted for in assessing renal disease.

      b) UTIs may be difficult to diagnose because some of the main symptoms (e.g., fever, pain) may not appear, may be less apparent, or may appear late in the elderly client.

      c) In the presence of a UTI, elderly clients may exhibit confusion and behavior changes as blood is diverted from the brain to the infection site. Development of incontinence may also signal UTI.

      d) Elderly clients may have misconceptions about sexuality. Reassure aging clients that despite normal changes in sexual response cycle, sexual activity can be continued and enjoyed.

      e) Discuss with aging clients the importance of performing regular breast self-exams and of having regular mammograms or prostate exams; provide client education in self-exam procedures.

1. As part of the general screening for gastrointestinal (GI) function, the nurse should evaluate the elderly client's swallowing reflex by:
   a. Touching the soft palate with a tongue blade and watching for gagging.
   b. Asking the client to swallow while palpating the esophagus for peristaltic waves.
   c. Watching the client eat and observing for signs of aspiration.
   d. Depressing the tongue and noting whether the soft palate rises when the client says "ah."

2. Which of the following observations related to the client's weight would support a diagnosis of malnutrition?
   a. Loss of 5% of the client's weight in 6 months
   b. Weight that is 10% over the ideal for the client
   c. Weight that is 10% below the ideal for the client
   d. Weight that is 5% below the ideal for the client

3. In order to provide sufficient dietary calcium for the elderly client who must avoid milk products to reduce symptoms of lactose intolerance, the nurse should advise increasing intake of which of the following?
   a. Green leafy vegetables
   b. Citrus fruits
   c. Red meats
   d. Whole grain breads

4. The elderly client with a hiatal hernia is most likely to report which symptom?
   a. Projectile vomiting
   b. Crampy lower abdominal pain
   c. Burning substernal pain
   d. Diarrhea

5. The elderly client who has recovered from acute diverticulitis should be taught to avoid:
   a. Orange juice and grapefruit juice.
   b. Cruciferous vegetables.
   c. Butter and cream.
   d. Sesame or poppy seed rolls.

6. When an elderly client is receiving cimetidine (Tagamet), it is important that the nurse monitor for which adverse effect?
   a. Chest pain
   b. Agitation
   c. Dyspnea
   d. Urinary retention

7. Which of the following is appropriate in planning a bladder training program for an incontinent elderly client?
   a. Having the client drink a full glass of water 30 minutes before each scheduled toileting time
   b. Toileting the client every 4 hours, even if he/she has been incontinent
   c. Giving no fluids after 8:00 P.M. except for small amounts with medications if required
   d. Serving hot beverages 30 minutes before each scheduled toileting time

8. Which of the following indicates that the client needs further teaching about Kegel exercises?
   a. The client tenses the pubococcygeal muscle, simulating the stopping of urine flow for 3 seconds.
   b. The client tenses the pubococcygeal muscle, buttocks, and thighs.
   c. The client performs the exercises in a sitting position.
   d. The client performs the exercises 4 times a day.

9. Which of the following may indicate urinary tract infection (UTI) in an elderly client?

   a. Development of incontinence
   b. Crampy abdominal pain
   c. Pale yellow urine
   d. Difficulty starting or maintaining the urine stream

10. Which of the following factors would increase the risk of vaginitis in an elderly client?

    a. Urinary incontinence
    b. Remaining sexually active
    c. Douching with vinegar
    d. Prolonged corticosteroid therapy

11. Which of the following would be a common nursing diagnosis for the client with benign prostatic hypertrophy?

    a. Sleep pattern disturbance
    b. Stress incontinence
    c. Constipation
    d. Pain

12. Which of the following test results is most likely to be misleading in relation to renal function in an elderly client?

    a. Elevated blood urea nitrogen (BUN)
    b. Impaired creatinine clearance
    c. Glycosuria on urinalysis
    d. Elevated specific gravity

ANSWERS

---

1. **Correct answer is d.** An important indicator of adequate swallowing function is the rising of the soft palate to block the nasopharynx.

   a. The gag reflex is a part of adequate swallowing function, but inducing gagging is uncomfortable and unnecessary since there are less unpleasant testing methods.
   b. This would not provide useful information about the adequacy of swallowing.

c. This is a valuable ongoing assessment, but providing a meal during the initial screening assessment would not be practical.

2. **Correct answer is c.** Criteria reflecting malnutrition include weight that is 10% below the client's ideal and loss of 5% of total body weight in 1 month.

   a. Loss of 10% of the client's weight in 6 months reflects malnutrition.
   b. Weight that is 20% over ideal is considered an indication of malnutrition.
   d. Although this might signal a need for monitoring, the client is not considered malnourished until he/she is 10% below the ideal weight.

3. **Correct answer is a.** Green leafy vegetables and dried beans are good sources of calcium.

   b, c, and **d.** None of these foods is high in calcium.

4. **Correct answer is c.** Heartburn, which is a burning substernal pain, is the most common sign of hiatal hernia in clients who experience any symptoms.

   a. Projectile vomiting is more likely to be associated with pyloric obstruction due to scarring from chronic peptic ulcer disease. Regurgitation would be a sign of hiatal hernia.
   b. Crampy pain in the lower abdomen is commonly associated with lactose intolerance.
   d. Diarrhea is more likely to be associated with diverticulitis.

5. **Correct answer is d.** Clients with diverticulitis need to avoid foods with kernels, nuts, or seeds (e.g., corn, tomatoes, foods garnished with seeds or nuts). Kernels or seeds may become lodged in diverticular pouches causing inflammation.

   a. Highly acidic juices should be avoided by clients with ulcers, gastritis, or hiatal hernia. They are not problematic for clients with diverticulitis.

b. Cruciferous vegetables, such as cabbage, broccoli, and cauliflower, are good sources of fiber for the client with diverticulosis or diverticulitis. The American Cancer Society recommends increasing these vegetables to decrease risk of colon cancer.

c. Butter and cream should be avoided by the client who needs a low-cholesterol diet. Cholesterol is not significant in the pathophysiology of diverticulitis.

6. **Correct answer is b.** Drowsiness, agitation, confusion, or mood swings may signal dangerous effects of cimetidine.

   a. Chest pain is more likely to reflect heartburn, which is a symptom that cimetidine is given to relieve.

   c. Dyspnea is a sign of an anaphylactic allergic reaction to any drug. It is not specific to cimetidine. Allergies to cimetidine are uncommon.

   d. Urinary retention is associated with drugs that have anticholinergic effects. Cimetidine is not likely to produce this effect.

7. **Correct answer is a.** The client should be toileted every 2 hours. Approximately 30 minutes before each toileting time, the client should be instructed to drink a full glass of water and make a conscious effort to retain the urine until the scheduled toileting time.

   b. Four hours is too long to wait between toileting times for an incontinent client who is beginning bladder training. If the usual time of 2 hours between scheduled times for toileting proves to be too long initially, the interval should be shortened.

   c. Limiting fluid intake is controversial. Concentrated urine causes urgency and may interfere with bladder training. Some experts recommend reducing the amount of fluid taken after 8:00 P.M., but completely withholding fluid would be inappropriate.

   d. Serving hot beverages is appropriate in a bowel training regimen, since it stimulates peristalsis and may induce defecation. It is not useful in bladder training.

8. **Correct answer is b.** Kegel exercises are most effective if the client does not tense buttock and thigh muscles. Since this client is not performing the exercises in the most effective manner, further teaching is indicated.

   a, c, and **d.** No additional teaching is needed. The pubococcygeal muscle alone is tensed in Kegel exercises. To help clients identify the correct muscle to tense, they are often told to simulate stopping the flow of urine; however, it is inappropriate to actually stop urinary flow while voiding, since this can lead to urinary tract infection (UTI). Kegel exercises are equally effective in a standing, sitting, or lying position. A series of 10 "squeezes" should be performed 3 or 4 times daily.

9. **Correct answer is a.** The urgency or frequency produced by UTI often causes incontinence in the elderly.

   b. Perineal, suprapubic, or low back pain are associated with UTI. Crampy abdominal pain is usually related to an intestinal problem.

   c. Pale yellow urine indicates adequate hydration. With UTI the urine may become pink or red (hematuria). Cloudy urine is also associated with UTI.

   d. Difficulty starting or maintaining a urine stream reflects prostatic hypertrophy. Burning or pain upon urination or urgency or frequency would be associated with UTI.

10. **Correct answer is d.** Because corticosteroids suppress immune system function, they increase the risk of inflammation produced by overgrowth of normal flora.

    a. No connection between incontinence and vaginitis has been reported.

    b. The risk of STDs is increased in sexually active clients. The most common causes of vaginitis in the elderly are overgrowth of normal flora and drying of vaginal mucosa.

    c. Acid douches, such as vinegar solution, are prescribed to treat vaginitis.

11. **Correct answer is a.** Because the bladder does not empty completely, nocturia may develop, causing the client to awaken frequently during the night.

b. Urinary retention may produce overflow incontinence. Stress incontinence is not normally associated with benign prostatic hypertrophy.

c. Although the enlarged prostate is palpable on rectal exam, prostatic enlargement is not usually sufficient to interfere with passage of stool.

d. Benign prostatic hypertrophy is not normally painful.

12. **Correct answer is c.** Abnormalities in urine glucose test results are common in the elderly and do not necessarily reflect renal function accurately.

a and **b.** Abnormalities of BUN and creatinine clearance are not uncommon in the elderly, but when found they accurately reflect altered renal function.

d. Urine specific gravity results are not influenced by the aging process.

9

Musculoskeletal and Integumentary Disorders

NURSING HIGHLIGHTS

1. Gradual loss of bone after age 40 is universal; loss is greater in women (about 25%) than in men (about 12%), leading to increased prevalence of osteoarthritis, osteoporosis, and fractures with age.
2. Diet, hormonal changes, and physical activity affect the rate of bone loss.
3. The nurse should provide support for clients who have arthritis as they deal with chronic pain, alterations in physical appearance, and role changes within the family.
4. The nurse should promote mobility among impaired elderly clients to the extent possible because of the high risk of the development of pressure sores and other losses of skin integrity.

GLOSSARY

cancellous bone tissue—spongy bone tissue
cortical bone tissue—compact bone tissue
crepitus—a continuous grating of a joint during movement
ecchymosis (pl. ecchymoses)—a hemorrhagic spot on the skin that is larger than a petechia; a bruise
osteotomy—cutting of a bone to promote realignment
pannus—vascular granular tissue, composed of inflammatory cells, that erodes cartilage and destroys bone
petechia (pl. petechiae)—a minute red spot on the skin that is caused by a small hemorrhage
synovitis—inflammation of the synovial membranes of the joints

ENHANCED OUTLINE

See text pages

_____

I. Musculoskeletal disorders

A. Age-related changes (see section II,F of Chapter 2)

B. General nursing assessment
1. General observation
   a) Observe the client for signs of functional disorders (e.g., abnormal gait); favoring 1 leg; indicators of paralysis, weakness, or musculoskeletal pain; and the use of an assistive device.
   b) Observe the client for the presence of structural abnormalities (e.g., an atrophied limb; red, swollen, deformed joints).
2. Interview
   a) Inquire about the presence of pain or functional impairment in any part of the body.
   b) Ask the client about a personal or family history of musculoskeletal disease (e.g., arthritis, osteoporosis).
   c) Find out whether the client has ever broken a bone, had a serious accident, participated intensively in athletics or gymnastics, or worked in an occupation that stresses the joints (e.g., construction, landscaping).
   d) Determine whether the client takes medication for musculoskeletal pain (e.g., ibuprofen); if so, ask the name of the pain reliever and how often it is taken.
3. Physical exam
   a) Examine the active and passive range of motion of all joints.
   b) Note any crepitus that is detected during movement.
   c) Assess for the presence of tremor, spasm, tightness, contracture, and abnormal muscular weakness.
   d) Assess for the presence of ataxia (e.g., failure of muscular coordination, erratic muscular function).

C. Common disorders
1. Osteoporosis
   a) Definition: metabolic disorder characterized by bone demineralization and decreased density that may lead to fractures, especially of the wrist, hip, and vertebral column
   b) Pathophysiology and etiology
      (1) Pathophysiology: decrease in calcium content of cancellous and cortical bone, leading to reduced bone mass

(2) Etiology
- (a) Primary osteoporosis: aging; decreased serum estrogen levels in postmenopausal women; insufficient consumption of calcium, vitamin D, and protein; small body frame; inactivity; immobility
- (b) Secondary osteoporosis: administration of anticonvulsants, corticosteroids, and heparin; bone cancer; cirrhosis; Cushing's syndrome; diabetes mellitus; hyperthyroidism; rheumatoid arthritis

c) Symptoms: hip, wrist, or vertebral fracture, often associated with minor trauma; kyphosis of the dorsal spine ("dowager's hump"); reduction in height; back pain that is aggravated by activity; voluntary restriction of spinal movement

d) Treatment: high-protein diet; administration of calcium and vitamin D supplements, sodium fluoride, and estrogen; administration of conjugated estrogen to postmenopausal women; avoidance of alcohol, caffeine, and smoking; range-of-motion exercises; prevention of falls

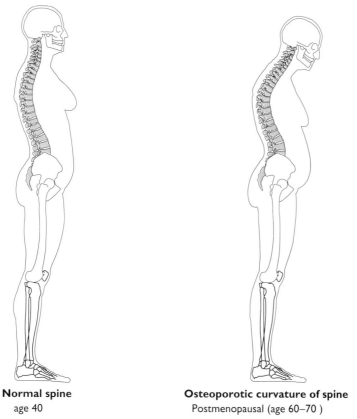

Normal spine
age 40

Osteoporotic curvature of spine
Postmenopausal (age 60–70)

Figure 9–1
Osteoporotic Changes in the Spine of the Elderly Woman

2. Fractures
   a) Definition: a break in the continuity of a bone
   b) Pathophysiology and etiology
      (1) Pathophysiology: age-related bone atrophy and demineralization often leading to a fracture of the neck of the femur, especially in elderly women
      (2) Etiology: problems of coordination, vision, hearing, balance, and cognition that increase the risk of falls; disorders that weaken bone structure (e.g., osteoporosis, bone cancer)
   c) Symptoms: pain, limited limb movement, change in limb length or shape, tissue spasm, edema, discoloration, protruding bone
   d) Treatment: casting, closed reduction, open reduction, traction, external fixation, total joint replacement
3. Osteoarthritis
   a) Definition: degenerative joint disease usually affecting weight-bearing joints and fingers
   b) Pathophysiology and etiology
      (1) Pathophysiology: steady deterioration and loss of articular cartilage in peripheral and axial joints; hypertrophy of bone at margins; reduced elasticity of the joint capsule, cartilage, and ligaments; narrowing of joint space
      (2) Etiology: degenerative process of aging; excessive use of 1 or more joints due to obesity, participation in athletics, or an occupation that causes stress to the joints; previous trauma
   c) Symptoms: progressive joint pain especially after use, crepitus, stiffness, bony nodes, functional impairment, secondary synovitis
   d) Treatment: analgesic for pain; nonsteroidal anti-inflammatory drugs (NSAIDs) for pain and for secondary inflammation; local, systemic, and psychologic rest; therapeutic exercise; maintenance of joints in their functional position; application of heat; diet high in protein and vitamin C; use of appropriate assistive and adaptive devices; surgery to correct immobility or relieve extreme pain
4. Rheumatoid arthritis
   a) Definition: an inflammatory disease that is chronic, progressive, and systemic; its primary effect is on the synovial joints
   b) Pathophysiology and etiology
      (1) Pathophysiology: thickening of synovium; accumulation of fluid in joint spaces; pannus formation; development of fibrous adhesions, bony ankylosis, calcifications, and secondary osteoporosis
      (2) Etiology: autoimmune abnormalities, genetic predisposition, hormonal imbalance, physical and emotional stress

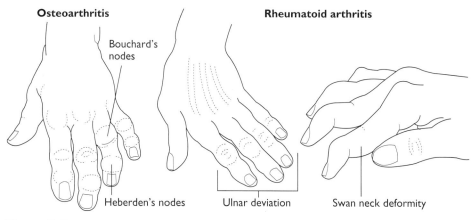

Osteoarthritis

Bouchard's nodes

Heberden's nodes

Rheumatoid arthritis

Ulnar deviation

Swan neck deformity

Figure 9–2
Common Arthritic Joint Deformities

    c) Symptoms
        (1) Early stage: fatigue; weakness; anorexia; small weight loss; persistent low-grade fever; joints that are warm, red, stiff, swollen and painful
        (2) Late stage: progressive pain and morning stiffness, joint deformities, anemia, fibrotic lung disease, osteoporosis, pericarditis, peripheral neuropathy, renal disease, severe fatigue, subcutaneous nodules, vasculitis, weight loss
    d) Treatment: administration of analgesics, antipyretics, and anti-inflammatory drugs; rest; joint positioning; therapeutic exercise; application of heat or cold; stress management; physical and occupational therapy; use of assistive and adaptive devices; surgery (e.g., synovectomy, osteotomy, total joint replacement)

D. Essential nursing care
  1. Nursing assessment (see section I,B of this chapter)
  2. Nursing diagnoses
    a) High risk for injury related to minor accidents
    b) Pain related to bone fracture
    c) Impaired physical mobility related to treatment of bone fracture
    d) Pain related to cartilage disruption
    e) Impaired physical mobility related to pain or deformity
    f) Self-esteem disturbance related to joint deformity and immobility
  3. Nursing implementation (intervention)
    a) Educate the client with osteoporosis in ways to avoid fractures associated with minor accidents (e.g., eliminating environmental hazards in the home such as throw rugs, performing activities of daily living [ADLs] cautiously).
    b) Provide pain-control measures related to a bone fracture.
        (1) Report a cast or bandage that is too tight.
        (2) Report when traction equipment does not relieve pain.

     (3) Administer prescribed analgesics and sedatives.

     (4) Supplement medication with other pain-control techniques (e.g., hot tea, music therapy, guided imagery).

   c) For a client with a fracture, provide measures to avoid complications related to immobility.

     (1) Monitor fluids.

     (2) Provide assistance with turning in bed.

     (3) Help the client ambulate as soon as possible. If the client is unable to walk, have the client bear weight during transfer from bed to chair.

     (4) Encourage coughing and deep breathing.

     (5) Administer anticoagulants as ordered.

     (6) Apply antiembolism stockings.

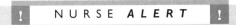

!   N U R S E   *A L E R T*   !

Side Effects of NSAIDs in the Elderly

The elderly are at increased risk for many of the side effects of anti-inflammatory drugs, notably NSAIDs, because of reduced hepatic and renal clearance rates and because of drug interactions. Monitor for these adverse side effects:

For all NSAIDs

- Tinnitus
- Blurred vision
- Gastric irritation
- Gastric bleeding leading to perforated ulcers
- Nausea
- Fluid retention, edema
- Reduced renal function

Penicillamine

- Hematologic side effects (e.g., aplastic anemia, leukopenia)
- Susceptibility of skin to injury on pressure points

Indomethacin: contraindicated with liver disease, kidney disease, active ulcer

- Central nervous system (CNS) side effects (e.g., confusion, tinnitus)

Phenylbutazone: given as a last resort in a 1-week dose with complete blood count (CBC) monitored

- Agranulocytosis
- Aplastic anemia

NOTE: Salicylates (e.g., aspirin) should not be given with other types of NSAIDs as they interfere with their actions.

Suggestions for Protecting the Joints

To reduce pain and prevent the acceleration of joint damage, the client with osteoarthritis, rheumatoid arthritis, or a related disorder should be given the following suggestions:

✔ Use the large joints of your body rather than the small ones. Use a purse with a shoulder strap rather than a hand strap.
✔ Hold heavy objects, such as pans, with 2 hands.
✔ Do not wring or twist your hands when doing household chores.
✔ Turn doorknobs counterclockwise instead of clockwise to prevent ulnar deviation.
✔ Bend at the knees rather than at the waist.
✔ Use a small pillow under your head when you are in bed. Otherwise, avoid the use of pillows as they may cause flexion contractures.
✔ When you get out of bed, push off with the palms of your hands rather than your fingers.
✔ Make daily activities less painful by using assistive and adaptive devices (e.g., clothing with Velcro fasteners, utensils with built-up handles).
✔ Sit in a straight chair with a high back.

(7) Encourage the use of isotonic and isometric exercises taught in physical therapy.

(8) Reinforce client teaching given in physical therapy about safe transfer from a bed or wheelchair and proper use of assistive devices (e.g., walker, cane).

d) Monitor the client who is taking NSAIDs or other antiarthritic drugs for adverse or toxic effects. Dosages may have to be lower due to lower clearance rates, especially among the impaired elderly (see Nurse Alert, "Side Effects of NSAIDs in the Elderly").

e) Instruct the client with osteoarthritis or rheumatoid arthritis in the proper use of appropriate medication (e.g., to use analgesics prior to performing ADLs or exercise).

f) Encourage the client with arthritis to follow the prescribed schedule of physical and occupational therapy and exercise and to take care when performing ADLs (see Client Teaching Checklist, "Suggestions for Protecting the Joints").

g) Confirm that the client with arthritis understands the need for and the proper use of assistive and adaptive devices.

h) Encourage the client experiencing a self-esteem disturbance because of joint deformity and immobility to take steps to maintain his/her physical appearance; participate to tolerance in family and social activities; and seek professional help for depression, sexual, family, or occupational problems.

4. Nursing evaluation
   a) The client with osteoporosis avoids fractures.
   b) The client with a fracture reports that pain has been alleviated or lessened.
   c) The client with a broken bone avoids complications associated with immobility and uses assistive devices to ambulate safely.
   d) The client with arthritis states that pain is tolerable.
   e) The client with arthritis maintains or increases physical mobility.
   f) The client with arthritis reports an improvement in self-esteem.
5. Gerontologic nursing considerations
   a) Elderly people with osteoporosis, who are at heightened risk of fall-related fractures, may be receiving medications for other conditions that increase their likelihood of falling. The nurse should monitor the client receiving diuretics, phenothiazines, or tranquilizers for adverse effects that might lead to falls.
   b) Fractures in older persons are associated with a high risk of serious or life-threatening complications, such as contractures, fecal impaction, pneumonia, pressure sores, renal calculi, and thrombus formation.
   c) Because the typical symptoms of a fracture may not be evident in elderly clients, each time they fall or suffer a trauma, they should be evaluated for fracture.
   d) Rheumatoid arthritis affects many age groups but the elderly have significant systemic symptoms (e.g., fatigue, malaise, weakness, weight loss, anemia, peripheral neuropathy).
   e) Arthritis and fractures compound the gait and balance problems associated with old age. The nurse should work with the physical therapist to make sure that clients use assistive devices properly and know how to get out of bed and chairs safely.

See text pages

II. Integumentary disorders

A. Age-related changes (see section II,G of Chapter 2)

B. General nursing assessment
   1. General observation
      a) Observe the general condition of the client's skin, including color, moisture, and cleanliness.
      b) Inspect the nails for signs of brittleness and discoloration.
      c) Note the cleanliness and overall condition of the hair.
      d) Take note of indicators of the general nutritional status.
      e) Take particular note of signs of underlying disease (e.g., pallor, flushing, lesions).

2. Interview
   a) Determine the history of the client's skin problem and ask whether it is associated with itching, pain, or burning.
   b) Ascertain the client's overall health status and the personal and family history of significant skin problems.
   c) Inquire about prescription and over-the-counter (OTC) drugs that the client has used recently.
   d) Ask whether the client has any known allergies.
   e) Inquire about the client's dietary habits, alcohol consumption, and tobacco use.
   f) Determine the client's occupation and leisure-time activities.
3. Physical exam
   a) Examine all skin surfaces, including the hair, scalp, nails, and mucous membranes.
   b) Note the color, texture, moisture, and integrity of the skin.
   c) Document the presence of skin lesions and edema.

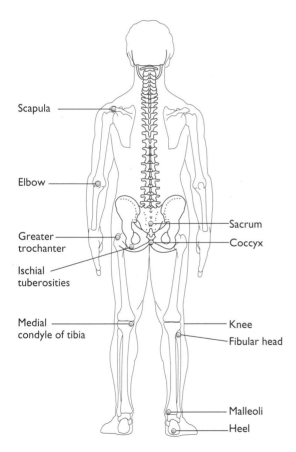

Figure 9–3
Bony Prominences That Are Main Sites of Pressure Sores

        d) Note the presence of normal skin markings (e.g., birthmarks, cherry and spider angiomas) and of abnormal markings (e.g., ecchymoses, petechiae).

        e) Palpate the skin to determine temperature, turgor, texture, and moisture.

   C. Common disorders

     1. Pressure sores

       a) Definition: an area of cellular necrosis, often over a bony prominence; also called decubitus, bedsore, pressure ulcer

       b) Pathophysiology and etiology

         (1) Pathophysiology: compression of skin and underlying tissue between bone and an underlying firm surface, leading to ischemia and anoxia

         (2) Etiology: immobility, poor nutritional status, extreme thinness, impaired sensory feedback mechanisms, corticosteroid therapy

       c) Symptoms

         (1) Stage 1 ulcer: area of unbroken skin that appears shiny with erythema over compressed area and that does not return to normal color after removal of pressure

         (2) Stage 2 ulcer: blistered or eroded areas of skin confined to the superficial epidermal and dermal layers

         (3) Stage 3 ulcer: broken skin creating a pressure sore that extends through all skin layers to affect underlying tissue

         (4) Stage 4 ulcer: deep pressure sore that involves muscle, bone, and joint tissues

       d) Treatment: diet high in proteins, carbohydrates, and vitamins; maintenance of moist wound environment with transparent film or hydrocolloid wafer dressings; control of drainage with Gelfoam, karaya powder, or absorption dressings; mechanical debridement with wet-to-dry dressings; chemical debridement; surgical debridement in severe cases

     2. Senile pruritus

       a) Definition: itching of the skin due to excessive dryness

       b) Pathophysiology and etiology

         (1) Pathophysiology: progressive loss of moisture in superficial skin tissues

         (2) Etiology: age-related atrophic changes, too-frequent or hot baths or showers, exposure to dry heat, stress, medication reaction, allergies, sudden temperature changes, arteriosclerosis, cancer, diabetes mellitus, liver disease, pernicious anemia, renal failure

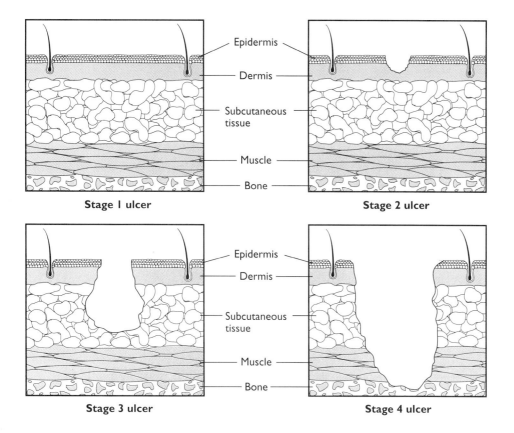

Figure 9–4
Stages of Skin Ulceration

     c) Symptoms: severe itching that can lead to traumatizing scratching that can cause skin breakage and infection

     d) Treatment: rehydration of the dermis with superfatted soaps, bath oils, lotions, and emollients; humidification of environment; cold saline compresses; Epsom salt or oatmeal baths; low bedtime doses of an antihistamine (e.g., hydroxyzine)

  3. Venous stasis ulcers

     a) Definition: ulcers developed due to an inadequacy of venous return from the legs with pooling of venous blood in the extremities

     b) Pathophysiology and etiology

        (1) Pathophysiology: weakening of the valves in the veins resulting in varicosities, edema of the lower extremities, poor tissue nutrition, and accumulation of debris and toxins

        (2) Etiology: genetic predisposition, prolonged standing, obesity, crossing of the legs

        c) Symptoms: edema; hyperpigmentation; stasis dermatitis; cracked skin; irregularly shaped skin ulcerations, usually on the ankles, that cause only minimal pain

        d) Treatment: bed rest; elevation of legs while sitting; compression with elastic bandages, antiembolism stockings, or support hose; application of topical antibiotics, normal saline solution, or Burow's compresses or soaks to stasis ulcers; chemical or surgical debridement; intermittent sequential compression boots

    4. Keratoses

        a) Definition: gray or brown horny growths that may be benign (seborrheic keratoses) or premalignant (actinic or solar keratoses)

        b) Pathophysiology and etiology

           (1) Pathophysiology: changes in the keratinocytes of the dermis leading to lesions that appear spontaneously

           (2) Etiology: prolonged exposure to the sun

        c) Symptoms

           (1) Seborrheic keratoses: wartlike projections that are dark and oily in sebaceous areas of the body and dry and light in other areas and do not have swelling or redness around their base

           (2) Actinic keratoses: small gray or brown lesions with an irregular border and possibly a reddened and swollen base

        d) Treatment: removal with freezing agents, acids, electrodesiccation, surgical excision

    5. Skin cancer

        a) Definition: cutaneous malignancy

        b) Pathophysiology and etiology

           (1) Pathophysiology

               (a) Squamous cell carcinomas: neoplasms of the epidermis in which there is local invasion and the potential for metastasis

               (b) Basal cell carcinomas: neoplasms that arise in the basal layer of the epidermis; rarely metastasize, but may invade underlying tissue (e.g., blood vessels, cartilage)

               (c) Melanomas: pigmented neoplasms that originate in the melanin-producing cells of the epidermis and are highly metastatic

           (2) Etiology: prolonged, excessive exposure to the sun; genetic predisposition; occupational exposure to arsenic and pesticides

        c) Symptoms

           (1) Squamous cell carcinomas: firm nodule that is topped with a crust or has an ulcerated area in the center; usually found on the head, neck, and lower lip

        (2) Basal cell carcinomas: pearly papule that has a central crater and waxy, rolled borders; usually found on the head, neck, and central portion of the face

        (3) Melanomas: irregularly shaped papule or plaque that is variegated with blue, red, and white tones; can appear anywhere on the body

    d) Treatment: drug therapy, radiation therapy, cryosurgery, curettage, electrodesiccation, excision

D. Essential nursing care

  1. Nursing assessment (see section II,B of this chapter)

  2. Nursing diagnoses

    a) Impaired skin integrity related to immobility

    b) High risk for impaired skin integrity related to itching

    c) High risk for infection related to venous stasis

    d) High risk for injury related to precancerous keratoses

    e) Impaired skin integrity related to malignant skin lesions

    f) Anxiety related to cancer diagnosis

  3. Nursing implementation (intervention)

    a) See section I,B,1,b of Chapter 4 for nursing interventions to prevent pressure sores. Treat pressure sores with appropriate dressing or debridement (see section II,C,1,d of this chapter); provide postoperative care to clients who have undergone surgical debridement.

    b) For senile pruritus, provide appropriate lotions or compresses and baths (see section II,C,2,d of this chapter); administer low bedtime doses of medication as ordered.

    c) Instruct the client with senile pruritus to avoid scratching the skin, wearing clothing that rubs, taking hot or too-frequent baths or showers, and drying vigorously.

    d) Instruct the client with venous stasis ulcers to prevent infection by applying topical antibiotics and to control discomfort from stasis ulcers by keeping the legs elevated and applying normal saline solution or Burow's compresses or soaks to affected areas.

    e) Teach elderly clients to inspect their skin regularly for the presence of skin lesions and to have all lesions evaluated and, if necessary, removed.

    f) Encourage the client with suspected skin cancer to pursue treatment. Explain the expected side effects of therapy, and encourage the use of precautions that will minimize the risk of complications (e.g., postsurgical infection).

    g) Encourage the client with skin cancer to discuss fears. Answer questions completely, and refer the client as needed to an appropriate counseling service.

  4. Nursing evaluation

    a) The immobile client with pressure sores regains skin integrity and avoids further ulceration.

    b) The client with senile pruritus maintains intact skin.

       c) The client with venous stasis ulcers avoids infection.

       d) The client with actinic keratoses has lesions removed prior to progression to squamous cell carcinoma.

       e) The client with skin cancer maintains skin integrity and avoids treatment-related complications.

       f) The client with skin cancer reports that anxiety has been reduced.

5. Gerontologic nursing considerations: A lifetime of occupational and recreational exposure to the sun may lead to the development of a variety of precancerous or cancerous lesions on the skin of older people.

1. Which of the following assessments is most suggestive of osteoporosis in an elderly woman?

    a. Joint pains that increase with use
    b. Joint stiffness in the morning
    c. Ataxic gait
    d. Back pain aggravated by activity

2. To reduce the risk of fractures, the elderly client should be instructed to step down from the sidewalk to the street by:

    a. Placing the toes of both feet against the curb's edge before stepping down with one foot.
    b. Keeping one foot at least 6 inches behind the curb's edge while stepping down with the other foot.
    c. Turning sideways so that he/she steps down by moving one foot to the side.
    d. Locating a sign post or utility pole to hold onto while stepping down.

3. Appropriate advice for the client with osteoarthritis would include:

    a. Application of ice to relieve joint inflammation.
    b. Increasing weight-bearing activities.
    c. Supporting joints in correct alignment while resting.
    d. Using analgesics only when pain is not relieved by rest.

4. In addition to discussing measures to control pain and maintain mobility, the nurse should teach the client with rheumatoid arthritis about:

    a. Stress management.
    b. Dietary changes to promote weight loss.
    c. Prevention of fluid volume excess.
    d. Use of calcium supplements.

5. The client receiving ibuprofen (Motrin) or other nonsteroidal anti-inflammatory drugs (NSAIDs) to control arthritic pain should be monitored for:

    a. Jaundice.
    b. Stomatitis.
    c. Diarrhea.
    d. Pedal edema.

6. Which of the following would be an appropriate suggestion for the nurse to give the client with rheumatoid arthritis?

    a. Avoid shoulder straps on purses.
    b. Turn doorknobs only clockwise.
    c. Avoid wringing movements of the hands.
    d. Use 2 pillows to elevate the head in bed.

7. Which of the following is a common site for the development of pressure ulcers?

    a. Buttocks over gluteus maximus
    b. Back over scapula
    c. Skin folds of groin
    d. Chest over the sternum

8. To relieve the itching from senile pruritus, the nurse should suggest:

    a. Warm compresses.
    b. Tepid oatmeal baths.
    c. Rubbing the skin with a towel.
    d. Applications of rubbing alcohol.

9. Assessments commonly associated with venous stasis ulcers include:

    a. Location on the sole of the foot.
    b. Regularly shaped ulceration.
    c. Hyperpigmented skin around the ulcer.
    d. Severe pain.

10. To promote healing of venous stasis ulcers, the nurse should suggest that the client:

    a. Raise the head of the bed on 6-inch blocks.
    b. Keep the legs elevated on a footstool while sitting.

c. Avoid wearing elastic stockings or support hose over the ulcer.

d. Perform Homans' maneuver at least 3 times daily.

11. The nurse should recognize which of the following as a risk factor for skin cancers?

a. Outdoor occupation, such as farming or forestry

b. High-fat diet

c. Exposure to secondhand smoke

d. Frequent home permanents

12. When teaching the client to recognize and report lesions that may be cancerous, the nurse should include which of the following characteristics?

a. Irregularly shaped blue papules

b. Small, flat red spots

c. Dark, oily, wartlike projections

d. Reddened areas with blistered surfaces

ANSWERS

1. **Correct answer is d.** Symptoms of osteoporosis include height reduction, kyphosis, and back pain aggravated by movement.

   a. Joint pain that worsens with movement is more often associated with osteoarthritis.
   b. Morning joint stiffness is more commonly associated with rheumatoid arthritis.
   c. Ataxic gait reflects spinal cord or cerebellar disease and is not associated with osteoporosis.

2. **Correct answer is a.** Standing with both feet at the edge of the curb and stepping down with one foot allows the center of balance to shift only slightly as the client steps down, reducing the risk of loss of balance and falling.

   b. Keeping one foot 6 inches behind the curb while stepping down with the other foot would require a longer stretch of the leg, producing poor balance during the downward step.

c. A lateral shift of balance combined with the step down throws the client off balance, increasing the risk of a fall.
d. It is not necessary to hold onto or lean against an object while stepping down as long as adequate precautions to maintain balance are taken.

3. **Correct answer is c.** Correct body alignment is important to maintain joints in functional positions. Keeping extremities in good alignment permits the joint to rest.

   a. Heat is prescribed to relieve aching and stiffness of joints. Ice would not be beneficial and might actually worsen the discomfort. Cold applications are sometimes prescribed to reduce inflammation in rheumatoid arthritis.
   b. Exercise that involves weight bearing puts more stress on joints and speeds the progression of the pathology.
   d. Analgesics are often prescribed on a regular schedule to maintain pain control and permit the client to continue activities of daily living (ADLs).

4. **Correct answer is a.** As with any autoimmune disease, poor stress management can lead to exacerbations. Since chronic illness is often stressful for the client and family, stress management is an important aspect of teaching for the client with rheumatoid arthritis.

   b. Clients with rheumatoid arthritis often lose weight. Measures to promote weight loss would be more appropriate for clients with osteoarthritis.
   c. Fluid volume excess is not a common problem for clients with rheumatoid arthritis.
   d. Calcium supplementation is not useful in treating rheumatoid arthritis. This teaching would be more appropriate for the client with osteoporosis.

5. **Correct answer is d.** Peripheral or dependent edema occurs as a result of sodium and fluid retention induced by NSAIDs.

   a. Jaundice would occur with liver damage, which is not a common toxicity of NSAIDs. Renal toxicity is more common with NSAIDs.

b. Stomatitis is seen with methotrexate, an antineoplastic drug that may be used to suppress the autoimmune disease process in rheumatoid arthritis. It is also a common side effect of gold salts. It is not anticipated with NSAIDs.

c. Diarrhea is a common side effect of antigout drugs such as colchicine. It is not associated with NSAIDs.

6. **Correct answer is c.** Wringing or twisting motions of the hands are stressful to inflamed wrist and finger joints and may promote ulnar deviations.

    a. Shoulder straps are more desirable than hand straps. Whenever possible large joints or the trunk should be used rather than small joints.

    b. Doorknobs should be turned counterclockwise to prevent ulnar deviation.

    d. A single flat pillow should be used in bed. More pillows would promote flexion contractures of the neck.

7. **Correct answer is b.** Pressure ulcers usually form over bony prominences that compress tissue, depriving it of nutrients and oxygen.

    a. The gluteus maximus is a muscle. There is no bony prominence in this area of the buttocks.

    c. Excoriation and maceration are common in skin folds, but pressure ulcers do not develop in skin folds that are not over bony prominences.

    d. Elderly clients seldom lie prone for prolonged periods, so the sternal area is not subject to pressure ulcer formation. Changes in spinal curvature and respiratory function make the prone position uncomfortable for most elderly clients.

8. **Correct answer is b.** Oatmeal baths soothe the skin and help relieve the itching. Vasoconstriction stimulated by the tepid temperature also helps reduce itching.

    a. Vasodilation induced by warm compresses would increase itching.

    c. Rubbing with rough fabrics like terry cloth toweling may damage the skin and is likely to stimulate increased itching.

    d. The cause of senile pruritus is progressive loss of moisture from the surface layers of the skin. Alcohol is a drying agent that would worsen this pathologic process.

9. **Correct answer is c.** Hyperpigmentation (stasis dermatitis) around the ankles and lower calves is a common sign of chronic venous stasis, which is the cause of venous stasis ulcers.

    a. Trophic ulcers, which are associated with diabetic neuropathy, are most often found in this location. Venous stasis ulcers more often occur on the ankles.

    b and **d.** A regular shape and severe pain are characteristics of arterial ulcers, which occur with peripheral vascular disease. Venous stasis ulcers usually have irregular borders and generally cause only minimal pain.

10. **Correct answer is b.** Elevating the legs promotes venous circulation by eliminating the negative effects of gravity. This may reduce venous stasis.

    a. Raising the head of the bed would be recommended for clients with arterial insufficiency. Since it would cause dependency of the legs, it would worsen venous stasis.

    c. Antiembolism stockings and support hose would be recommended because they provide compression, which helps reduce edema and venous stasis, promoting healing of venous stasis ulcers.

    d. Homans' maneuver is performed to test for thromboembolism. It is not a therapeutic measure.

11. **Correct answer is a.** Prolonged or frequent exposure to sun is the primary risk factor for skin cancers.

    b. High-fat diets have been implicated in gastrointestinal (GI) and reproductive system cancers. No dietary risk factors for skin cancer have been identified.

c. Smoking and exposure to secondhand smoke produce the same risks, which include lung and bladder cancers. There is no evidence that smoke affects skin cancer risk. **d.** Some chemical exposures, such as pesticides, do increase skin cancer risk. There is no conclusive evidence that home permanents increase risk of skin cancer.

12. **Correct answer is a.** Irregularly shaped blue papules suggest melanoma, a very malignant type of skin cancer.

   b. Small, flat red spots describe petechiae, which are the result of small hemorrhages; they are not malignant.

   c. Dark, oily, wartlike projections describe seborrheic keratoses, which commonly appear with old age and are not cancerous.

   d. Reddened areas with blistered surfaces suggest a stage 2 pressure ulcer or allergic reaction, not a cancerous process.

10

Hematologic and Endocrine Disorders

NURSING HIGHLIGHTS

1. The nurse should be aware that a factor contributing to the occurrence of anemias in elderly people is the inability to pay for or prepare nutritious food. The nurse should be familiar with local agencies that may be able to help.
2. The nurse must tailor the care plan for the elderly client with diabetes to that person's capabilities in an attempt to offer as much independence as possible.
3. The nurse must be aware of the atypical situations that arise in the elderly client with diabetes. The elderly client presents differently from the younger person, and glucose levels are normally higher for older adults.

GLOSSARY

hypochromia—condition in which red blood cells are low in or devoid of pigment

intrinsic factor—substance secreted by the gastric mucosa; needed for absorption of cyanocobalamin (vitamin B_{12}) from intestinal tract

ENHANCED OUTLINE

I. Hematologic disorders

See text pages
_____

A. Age-related changes (see section IV,B,3,a-b of Chapter 2)

B. General nursing assessment
   1. General observation
      a) Observe skin for ecchymoses, pallor, dryness, or loss of tone.
      b) Observe the nails and hair for brittleness or thinness.
      c) Observe changes in mood or alertness (e.g., irritability, fatigue, depression, confusion).
   2. Interview
      a) Ask about any recent increase in fatigue.
      b) Ask about recent weight loss, loss of appetite, or occurrences of nausea or vomiting.
      c) Inquire about tenderness or pain near the liver, spleen, or lymph nodes.
   3. Physical examination
      a) Examine skin for pallor, petechiae, and ecchymoses.
      b) Examine the mucous membranes for pallor and ecchymoses.
      c) Check the tongue: Redness, smoothness, and atrophy may indicate pernicious anemia.
      d) Assess lymph nodes for enlargement.

C. Common disorders
   1. Iron deficiency anemia
      a) Definition: a condition in which iron levels in the body are inadequate to synthesize hemoglobin
      b) Pathophysiology and etiology
         (1) Pathophysiology: decrease in the number of red blood cells and in hemoglobin levels; hypochromic, microcytic red blood cells
         (2) Etiology: deficiency of dietary iron (usually the cause in the elderly), impaired iron absorption, blood loss (e.g., due to peptic ulcer, gastrointestinal tumor), underlying condition (e.g., chronic hepatitis, urinary tract or other chronic infection); exacerbated by alcoholism
      c) Symptoms: hemoglobin level below 12 g/dl; hematocrit value below 35%; serum iron concentration below 42 µg/dl; headache; dizziness; fatigue; dry, inelastic skin; thin, brittle hair; thin, brittle, easily broken fingernails; atrophy or soreness of the tongue

d) Treatment: iron supplements (e.g., ferrous sulfate, gluconate, fumarate), improved nutrition, correction of the underlying condition
2. Pernicious anemia
    a) Definition: a progressive anemia occurring primarily in the elderly in which production of red blood cells is decreased due to insufficient absorption of vitamin B_{12} from food
    b) Pathophysiology and etiology
        (1) Pathophysiology: absence of intrinsic factor in stomach cells, reduced platelet and white blood cell (WBC) counts, macrocytic red blood cells
        (2) Etiology: impaired absorption of vitamin B_{12}, dietary vitamin B_{12} deficiency (rare); may occur if ileum is diseased or removed through surgery; frequently associated with cancer of the stomach
    c) Symptoms: weakness; listlessness; pallor; nervousness; mild diarrhea; smooth, red tongue; numbness and tingling of hands and feet
    d) Treatment: weekly, then monthly vitamin B_{12} injections; periodic stool examination for evidence of stomach cancer
3. Folic acid deficiency anemia
    a) Definition: a condition in which folic acid levels in the body are inadequate to produce red blood cells
    b) Pathophysiology and etiology
        (1) Pathophysiology: inadequate DNA synthesis in precursor red blood cells leading to decrease in the number of mature red blood cells
        (2) Etiology: poor nutrition, possibly exacerbated by alcoholism, prolonged intravenous (IV) feeding, or total parenteral nutrition (TPN)
    c) Symptoms: pallor; smooth, red tongue; fatigue; weight loss
    d) Treatment: folic acid therapy, improved nutrition
4. Chronic leukemias
    a) Definition: malignancies of the hematopoietic system; chronic lymphocytic leukemia (CLL) occurs primarily in people over 50; chronic myelogenous leukemia (CML) has an increased incidence in people over 50
    b) Pathophysiology and etiology
        (1) Pathophysiology: abnormal, unregulated proliferation of immature white blood cells in the bone marrow preventing production of erythrocytes, platelets, and mature leukocytes; usually insidious onset
        (2) Etiology: age-related altered immune response and decreased size and response of lymphatics, possible genetic influence

c) Symptoms
   (1) Chronic lymphocytic leukemia: *may be asymptomatic in the elderly;* fatigue, activity intolerance, enlarged lymph nodes and spleen, anemia, infection, lymphocytosis, intermittent remissions and recurrences
   (2) Chronic myelogenous leukemia: *may be asymptomatic for years;* weakness, fatigue, bleeding, leukocytosis, pain from enlarged spleen
d) Treatment
   (1) Chronic lymphocytic leukemia: if mild, no treatment; chemotherapy
   (2) Chronic myelogenous leukemia: chemotherapy, bone marrow transplant

D. Essential nursing care
   1. Nursing assessment (same as section I,B of this chapter)
   2. Nursing diagnoses
      a) Activity intolerance related to fatigue
      b) Self-care deficit related to fatigue
      c) Altered nutrition, less than body requirements, related to anorexia, tongue atrophy or soreness, and/or fatigue
      d) Altered nutrition, less than body requirements, related to nausea and anorexia associated with chemotherapy
      e) High risk for infection related to reduction in immune function
      f) Body image disturbance related to hair loss associated with chemotherapy
   3. Nursing implementation (intervention)
      a) Ensure that the client receives sufficient rest.
      b) Assist the client with self-care and other activities as necessary until fatigue associated with anemia is alleviated.
      c) Encourage the client to improve nutrition; work with the client to establish a balanced diet with improved intake of vitamins and minerals.
         (1) For iron deficiency: red meat, liver, kidney beans, spinach, carrots, raisins
         (2) For folic acid deficiency: citrus fruits, leafy green vegetables, dried beans, nuts
      d) Protect the client with leukemia from the risk of infection.
         (1) Systematically monitor for signs of infection, which may be atypical in the elderly.
         (2) Wash hands frequently, and wear gloves during IV infusions.

     (3) Keep the client's supplies separate.

     (4) See that the client does not eat uncooked foods.

     (5) Limit the client's close contact with visitors.

     (6) To prevent skin infections, bathe the client daily and protect the client from skin abrasions and pressure sores.

     (7) Ensure normal elimination to prevent intestinal trauma.

     (8) Remove standing water (e.g., for fresh flowers or in denture cups) from the room.

  e) Encourage the client to choose attractive clothing and wig to maintain best personal appearance throughout chemotherapy.

4. Nursing evaluation

  a) The client indicates the ability to perform the activities of daily living (ADLs) without fatigue or asks for help when needed.

  b) The client's improved diet allows sufficient energy to attend to ADLs and self-care.

  c) The client stays free of significant infection.

  d) The client makes a positive adjustment to the temporary change in appearance during chemotherapy.

5. Gerontologic nursing considerations

  a) After age 71, normal iron values are 50%–75% of the values for younger adults.

  b) In many cases, hematologic disorders occur in the elderly because of financial constraints. Older people fearful of running through their resources will often skip or skimp on meals.

  c) A client who has trouble chewing or swallowing often eliminates red meat and fresh fruits from the diet, leading to anemias. Instruct the client in appropriate food preparation methods to ensure the proper intake of essential vitamins and minerals; also instruct the client that he/she should seek treatment of the cause of the chewing or swallowing problem.

  d) Assist the client in obtaining food stamps or help the client make contact with programs such as Meals on Wheels so that he/she does not cut back on essential nourishment.

  e) Be aware that the elderly client may not report symptoms of a hematologic disorder because he/she may assume symptoms such as fatigue, dyspnea on exertion, or pallor are normal signs of aging.

  f) Be aware of noncompliance issues related to vitamin B_{12} therapy and iron therapy, especially when symptoms disappear. Instruct the client that treatment must continue even after the client is feeling better.

  g) The elderly are at increased risk for the complications associated with leukemia. Risk of infection is increased due to reduced immune function, and hemorrhage can be very serious due to the reduced ability of the elderly to restore homeostasis.

See text pages
_____

II. Endocrine disorders

A. Age-related changes
   1. See section II,D of Chapter 2
   2. Reduced responses to stress due to:
      a) Decreased adrenocorticotropic hormone (ACTH) secretion
      b) Reduced adrenal secretion of norepinephrine and epinephrine
      c) Reduced secretion of glucocorticoids
      d) Heart rate that is slower to increase in response to stress and that, once elevated, takes longer to return to normal

B. General nursing assessment
   1. General observation
      a) Observe the client's overall appearance, paying particular attention to fat distribution and muscle mass.
      b) Note any signs of lethargy, depression, agitation, or nervousness.
      c) Check the skin for areas of discoloration or uneven pigmentation, bruising, petechiae, and vitiligo.
      d) Check for abnormal patterns of hair distribution, hirsutism, excessive hair loss, and unusual hair texture.
      e) Observe the client's nails for thickness or brittleness, which may be associated with thyroid disorders.

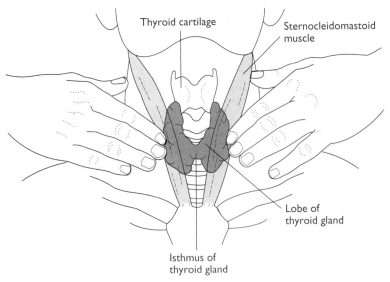

Figure 10–1
Palpation of the Thyroid Gland

2. Interview
    a) Ascertain whether there is a family history of obesity, growth disorders, diabetes, or thyroid disorders.
    b) Ask whether the client has noticed a recent change in energy level or the ability to perform everyday tasks.
    c) Inquire about elimination patterns, including urinary frequency and amount, nocturia, painful urination, frequency of bowel movements, and consistency and color of feces.
    d) Ask whether there has been any change in the client's nutritional status, including a recent increase or decrease in food and fluid intake.
    e) Determine whether the client has noticed any change in physical characteristics, such as hair color and distribution, facial contours, voice quality, and body proportions.
    f) Ask whether the client's tolerance for environmental heat or cold has decreased.
3. Physical examination
    a) Auscultate to determine vital signs and detect abnormalities of cardiac rate and rhythm.
    b) Note any difference in blood pressure and pulse when the client is lying down, sitting, and standing.
    c) Palpate the thyroid gland to determine its size, shape, and presence of nodules.

! NURSE *ALERT* !

Signs of Myxedema

Risk factors
- Long-term untreated hypothyroidism combined with:
  —Stress of illness
  —Exposure to cold
  —Trauma
  —Surgery
  —Hypnotic and sedative drugs

Symptoms
- Intense cold intolerance
- Subnormal pulse and temperature
- Expressionless face
- Drowsiness
- Personality changes (e.g., paranoid delusions)
- Profound lethargy
- Unconsciousness

Treatment
- Drug: immediate high doses of thyroid hormone
- Method: intravenous (IV) administration or injection

      d) Examine the extremities and base of the spine for edema, which may indicate fluid or electrolyte imbalance often associated with endocrine disorders.

      e) Examine the trunk for signs of adrenocortical excess, including truncal obesity, supraclavicular fat pads, buffalo hump, and reddish purple striae.

C. Common disorders

    1. Maturity-onset diabetes mellitus (also called type II diabetes or non-insulin-dependent diabetes mellitus)

      a) Definition: metabolic disorder of the pancreas in which insulin insufficiency or delayed release causes glucose intolerance

      b) Pathophysiology and etiology

         (1) Pathophysiology: age-related decreased glucose tolerance due to changes in insulin production and release and decreased affinity of receptor sites for insulin

         (2) Etiology: obesity, decreased exercise, increased fat tissue, decreased lean body mass, age-related physiologic and emotional stressors; may be secondary to pancreatic disease, use of medications (e.g., corticosteroids, thiazide diuretics)

      c) Symptoms: *asymptomatic or atypical in the elderly;* infection that heals slowly, orthostatic hypotension, arterial disease, gastric hypotony, impotence, neuropathy, confusion, glaucoma, Dupuytren contractures; some signs (e.g., blurred vision, weakness, fatigue, itching of the female genitalia) often taken for signs of aging or other disorders

      d) Treatment: insulin injections or oral hypoglycemic agents, diet, exercise, weight control

---

❗ NURSE *ALERT* ❗

Cautions with Thyroid Replacement Therapy in the Elderly Client

Low doses must be used at the start of thyroid replacement therapy for the elderly because of the possibility of aggravation of the following conditions:

- Angina
- Dysrhythmia
- Congestive heart failure
- Dementia
- Arteriosclerosis

2. Hypothyroidism
   a) Definition: insufficient thyroid hormone secretion
   b) Pathophysiology and etiology
      (1) Pathophysiology: metabolic rate decrease originating within thyroid (primary hypothyroidism) or pituitary (secondary hypothyroidism)
      (2) Etiology: autoimmune thyroiditis, thyroid gland atrophy
   c) Symptoms: *atypical in the elderly and often undiagnosed;* when seen, depression, apathy, decreased activity, psychomotor retardation; may advance to myxedema (see Nurse Alert, "Signs of Myxedema")
   d) Treatment: thyroid hormone replacement therapy (see Nurse Alert, "Cautions with Thyroid Replacement Therapy in the Elderly Client")
3. Impaired thermoregulation
   a) Definition: inability to maintain a consistent core body temperature of approximately 98.6°F (37°C) in an environment of extreme heat (hyperthermia) or cold (hypothermia)
   b) Pathophysiology and etiology
      (1) Pathophysiology: reduced ability to respond to extremes of environmental temperature, decreased cardiopulmonary reserves, impaired neurovascular response to extremes of temperature, inability to adjust basal metabolic rate

---

✔ CLIENT TEACHING CHECKLIST ✔

Preventing Hyperthermia

Discuss with elderly clients the following precautions they can take during prolonged hot and humid periods:

✔ Get adequate rest; avoid physical exercise, especially anything strenuous.
✔ Wear loose, lightweight, light-colored clothing.
✔ Increase fluid intake beyond what quenches the thirst.
   —Drink cool, nonalcoholic, noncaffeinated beverages.
✔ Increase salt intake only with the advice of a physician.
✔ Take cool-water baths.
✔ Keep your rooms at 75°F with the use of fans or air conditioners.
   —If you live in a high-crime area and keep all windows sealed during the summer, you must be especially careful to use fans or air conditioners.
   —If you cannot afford fans or air conditioners, go to places (e.g., shopping malls, senior citizen centers) that are air-cooled or contact churches or social service agencies that may be able to supply these items.
✔ Have someone look in on you regularly during a heat wave.

      (2) Etiology: cardiovascular, peripheral vascular, hematologic, and neurologic disorders; poor nutritional and fluid intake

         (a) Hyperthermia: effects of antihistamines, haloperidol, propranolol, diuretics, and phenothiazines; excessive activity in hot weather

         (b) Hypothermia: stress of surgery and effects of anesthetics; alcohol consumption; effects of hypnotics, barbiturates, benzodiazepines, antipsychotics; low level of activity in cold weather

   c) Symptoms

      (1) Hyperthermia: hot, dry skin; lack of perspiration; core temperature in excess of 104°F (40°C); dehydration; confusion; lethargy progressing to coma

      (2) Hypothermia: confusion, belligerence, disorientation, weakness, fatigue; core temperature of 95°F (34.9°C) or lower; shivering may or may not be evident

   d) Treatment

      (1) Hyperthermia: cool ambient environment, hydration with cool fluids, removal of excess clothing, treatment of underlying medical problems (see Client Teaching Checklist, "Preventing Hyperthermia")

✔ CLIENT TEACHING CHECKLIST ✔

Preventing Hypothermia

Most cases of hypothermia are preventable. Discuss the following cold-weather guidelines with elderly clients:

✔ Keep room temperatures 70°F or higher.

✔ If heat costs are too high, heat only the rooms you must use and remain there.

✔ Keep plenty of blankets on your bed and sleep with flannel sheets, a nightcap, socks, and warm pajamas.

✔ Wear layered clothing, with lighter clothing next to the skin and heavier garments on the outside. Wear a cap indoors on very cold days.

✔ Drink warm beverages and avoid alcohol consumption, especially near bedtime.

✔ If living alone, have a relative or neighbor call or look in every day.

✔ Contact your church or a local social service agency if you are concerned about paying your utility bills.

✔ Insulate areas around windows and doors through which cold air leaks. Local utilities or service agencies may provide weatherproofing at low or no cost.

(2) Hypothermia: warm ambient environment; cautious application of external warmth; warm, noncaffeinated fluids; removal of cold or wet clothing; mechanical ventilation and cardiopulmonary resuscitation (CPR) in severe cases; treatment of underlying medical problems (see Client Teaching Checklist, "Preventing Hypothermia"; see also section I,E,6 of Chapter 4 for preventing postoperative hypothermia)

D. Essential nursing care
  1. Nursing assessment (same as section II,B of this chapter)
  2. Nursing diagnoses
      a) Knowledge deficit related to self-care skills in diabetes
      b) Anxiety related to fear of complications or loss of independence
      c) High risk for infection related to vascular complications of diabetes
      d) Altered nutrition, more or less than body requirements, related to poor dietary control of diabetes
      e) Activity intolerance related to decreased energy levels associated with hypothyroidism
      f) High risk for altered body temperature related to hypothyroidism
      g) Hyperthermia resulting from high ambient temperatures and lack of air circulation in closed-up residence
      h) Hypothermia resulting from too-cool environment and insufficient nutrition
  3. Nursing implementation (intervention)
      a) Provide the elderly client who has diabetes with individualized client education about methods of promoting health and preventing injury, self-monitoring blood glucose, and self-administering insulin (see Client Teaching Checklist, "Self-Care for the Elderly Client with Diabetes").
      b) Reassure the client with diabetes that common complications (e.g., infections, neuropathies) can be minimized with good control.
      c) Teach the client with diabetes to recognize signs of infection; an early sign in the elderly may be mental status changes.
      d) Help the client establish an appropriate diet and exercise program suitable to the client's lifestyle.
      e) For the client with diabetes for whom financial difficulties or physical restraints might cause him/her to skip or skimp on meals, provide assistive devices or contact agencies to provide meals.
      f) Assist the client with hypothyroidism to perform self-care and hygiene activities; encourage him/her to perform as many activities as possible to prevent complications of immobility.
      g) Provide the client with cold intolerance with warm blankets and keep the client from drafts.
      h) Advise the elderly client at risk for impaired thermoregulation about resources for help with energy bills and appropriate clothing and activity levels during temperature extremes.

4. Nursing evaluation
    a) The client with diabetes demonstrates self-care skills and states an understanding of common diabetes complications and their management.
    b) The client with diabetes remains free from infection.
    c) The client with diabetes exercises daily and controls caloric intake.
    d) The client with hypothyroidism maintains an adequate level of activity and performs self-care measures as needed.
    e) The client with a thermoregulation problem maintains a core temperature in the range of 96°–99°F (37.2°–35.5°C).
    f) The elderly client makes appropriate environmental and behavioral modifications to avoid exposure to temperature extremes.
5. Gerontologic nursing considerations
    a) The older client with diabetes will find it difficult to change lifelong habits. Take into consideration the client's lifestyle when preparing a self-care plan.
    b) The elderly client with diabetes may worry about ability to carry out the treatment regimen and may need periodic reinforcement of education about medications, diet, and foot care and practice of self-care skills.

✔ CLIENT TEACHING CHECKLIST ✔

Self-Care for the Elderly Client with Diabetes

Explanation to the client:

✔ Have periodic follow-up examinations by the health care team.
✔ Report immediately any difficulty reading testing or medication labels or carrying out self-care measures.
✔ All insulins are different; do not borrow insulin from a friend.
✔ Do not follow fad diets or otherwise deviate from the recommended diet.
✔ Do not change your exercise program without notifying your health care provider. Slow, consistent exercise is the most effective.
✔ Foot care is critical to preventing infection. Report any problem immediately.
✔ Because many medications interfere with antidiabetic medications, report all medications that you are using.
✔ Report immediately signs of hypoglycemia.

c) The elderly client with diabetes may have problems with vision, mobility, memory, motor coordination, or other illnesses (e.g., arthritis, hypertension) that impede his/her ability to perform self-care measures and regulate blood glucose.

d) Arrange for the client who has self-care limitations to secure assistive devices such as a magnifying glass to read syringe markers or labels or an insulin pen. If necessary, get assistance from a visiting nurse or other community health group to arrange for insulin dispensing or glucose testing.

e) The elderly client with diabetes is at high risk for complications of the disease: hypoglycemia, which may cause falls; dehydration; infections of extremities (especially feet); and eye problems.

f) Hypoglycemia is a greater threat than ketoacidosis for older clients who have diabetes; signs, which may be atypical, include behavior disorders, poor sleep patterns, nocturnal headache, disorientation, confusion, and convulsions.

g) Diabetes testing results may be different in the elderly than in younger adults.
   (1) Fasting glucose level may be normal in older adults with diabetes.
   (2) Hyperglycemia may occur without glycosuria because older adults have an increased renal threshold for glucose.
   (3) Glucose tolerance tests to detect maturity-onset diabetes mellitus should allow 10 mg/dl above normal criteria for each decade beyond age 55.

h) In the elderly with hypothyroidism, special care must be taken with the administration of analgesics, sedatives, and anesthetics due to prolonged drug effects and reduced metabolic rate.

i) Heat stroke has a slower and subtler course in the elderly.

j) Advise elderly clients to keep their thermostat at 70°–88°F year-round. Financial difficulties and reduced perception of ambient temperatures may lead elderly clients to fail to heat and cool their homes adequately.

1. Which of the following nursing diagnoses is most appropriate for the client with iron deficiency anemia?

   a. Activity intolerance related to fatigue
   b. Altered nutrition, less than body requirements, related to tongue soreness
   c. High risk for infection related to low white blood cell (WBC) count
   d. Diarrhea related to side effects of iron therapy

2. Which of the following would be the most appropriate snack for the client with iron deficiency anemia?

   a. A half grapefruit
   b. A carrot raisin salad
   c. A cup of yogurt
   d. Apple slices and cheese

3. Which of the following assessment findings should alert the nurse to the possibility that an elderly client has pernicious anemia?

   a. Clubbing of the nails
   b. Bloody stools
   c. Smooth, beefy red tongue
   d. Enlarged lymph nodes

4. An elderly client who is being treated for pernicious anemia needs to be monitored periodically for:

   a. Lactose intolerance.
   b. Stomach cancer.
   c. Dementia.
   d. Hearing loss.

5. Which of the following would be the best lunch for a client with folic acid deficiency anemia?

   a. Bologna sandwich and vegetable soup
   b. Grilled cheese sandwich and tomato soup
   c. Coleslaw and cream of mushroom soup
   d. Spinach salad and bean soup

6. To reduce the risk of infection, the client with chronic myelogenous leukemia (CML) should be advised to:

   a. Have the water in flower arrangements changed frequently.
   b. Reduce the number of visitors.
   c. Bathe daily with mild soap.
   d. Avoid using lotions and creams.

7. The elderly client with non-insulin-dependent diabetes mellitus can improve blood sugar control by:

   a. Losing weight.
   b. Avoiding vigorous exercise.
   c. Reducing intake of complex carbohydrates.
   d. Increasing fluid intake.

8. The risk of non-insulin-dependent diabetes mellitus would be increased by which of the following medications?

   a. Dexamethasone (Decadron)
   b. Propranolol (Inderal)
   c. Ibuprofen (Motrin)
   d. Digoxin (Lanoxin)

9. The correct technique for examining the thyroid gland includes:

   a. Facing the client and grasping the gland between the thumb and forefinger of 1 hand.
   b. Standing behind the client and placing the fingertips of both hands against the sides of the gland.
   c. Palpating the anterior surface of the gland with the palm of 1 hand.
   d. Standing behind the client and placing 1 hand above and the other hand below the gland.

10. Thyroid hormone replacement therapy may aggravate which of the following conditions?

   a. Diabetes mellitus
   b. Anemia
   c. Renal failure
   d. Congestive heart failure (CHF)

11. During a heat wave, the nurse should advise elderly clients to:

   a. Increase their salt intake.
   b. Exercise in the late afternoon.
   c. Avoid caffeine.
   d. Wear dark clothing.

12. The elderly client's risk of hypothermia is increased by:

   a. Vigorous exercise.
   b. Moderate alcohol use.
   c. Hyperthyroidism.
   d. Nonsteroidal anti-inflammatory drugs (NSAIDs).

ANSWERS

1. **Correct answer is a.** Decreased oxygen transport due to low hemoglobin levels results in fatigue.

   b. Tongue soreness is associated with pernicious anemia, not iron deficiency.
   c. In anemias the red blood cell (RBC) count, not the WBC count, is decreased.
   d. Oral iron preparations cause constipation, not diarrhea.

2. **Correct answer is b.** Carrots and raisins are both high in iron. Red meats and spinach are other good iron sources.

   a. Citrus fruits are high in folic acid.
   c and d. Dairy products such as yogurt and cheese provide calcium, not iron. Fruits are generally not good sources of iron.

3. **Correct answer is c.** Early in the course of pernicious anemia the tongue becomes beefy red and painful. Later the tongue atrophies and becomes smooth.

   a. Nail clubbing is associated with respiratory and cardiac disorders. Numbness and tingling of the hands and feet are more common with pernicious anemia.
   b. Mild diarrhea is associated with pernicious anemia whereas bloody stools usually are not. Colorectal bleeding is likely to lead to iron deficiency anemia.
   d. Enlarged lymph nodes are associated with leukemia, not anemia.

4. **Correct answer is b.** The incidence of stomach cancer is increased in clients with deficiency of gastric acid (intrinsic factor). Treatment of pernicious anemia corrects the deficiency of vitamin B_{12} but does not alter the gastric acid production, so the client remains at risk for stomach cancer.

   a and d. Both lactose intolerance and hearing loss occur more commonly with aging, as does pernicious anemia. However, the presence of pernicious anemia does not alter the risk for either lactose intolerance or hearing loss.
   c. Dementia does occur in the late stages of untreated pernicious anemia, but for a client who is receiving treatment, there would be no increased risk of dementia.

5. **Correct answer is d.** Leafy green vegetables and dried beans are good sources of folic acid. Nuts and citrus fruits are other good sources.

   a, b, and c. These menus do not include any foods that are high in folic acid.

6. **Correct answer is c.** Daily bathing reduces the number of microorganisms on the skin, which reduces the risk of cutaneous infections.

   a. All standing water (in vases and denture cups) should be removed from the client's room.

b. It is not necessary to limit the number of visitors. The client should be advised to reduce close physical contact with visitors and to ask family and friends who have colds or "flu" not to visit.

d. Lotions and creams help restore moisture to the skin, reducing the risk of skin breakdown. It is important to avoid breaks in skin, which would permit entry of infecting organisms.

7. **Correct answer is a.** For some clients weight loss alone brings blood glucose levels into the normal range. Maintaining normal body weight improves glucose tolerance in all clients.

b. Exercise enables glucose to enter muscle cells even in the absence of insulin, reducing blood glucose levels. In the absence of cardiovascular complications, there is no contraindication to vigorous exercise in the client with diabetes mellitus.

c. Simple sugars should be avoided by the client with diabetes. The American Diabetes Association recommends increasing the proportion of complex carbohydrates in the diet.

d. Fluid intake may need to be increased to compensate for osmotic diuresis. It will not contribute to the control of blood glucose levels.

8. **Correct answer is a.** Corticosteroids, such as dexamethasone, raise blood glucose levels and impair glucose tolerance. Thiazide diuretics also increase the risk.

b. Beta blockers, such as propranolol, mask signs and symptoms of hypoglycemia in people with diabetes but do not increase the risk of diabetes mellitus.

c and d. Neither NSAIDs, such as ibuprofen, nor digoxin alter blood sugar levels or glucose tolerance.

9. **Correct answer is b.** The examiner stands behind the client and palpates the gland with the fingertips placed on either side of the gland. One hand can be used to displace the gland toward the other hand.

a. The thumb does not provide adequate examining surface for palpation. This position would not allow displacement of the gland.

c. The palm is not sufficiently sensitive to detect small nodules.

d. The gland cannot be displaced laterally using this position. Most of the gland is located lateral to the trachea, so this position would not provide contact with the majority of the gland's surface.

10. **Correct answer is d.** Cardiac disorders, such as angina, dysrhythmia, and CHF, are aggravated by the increased metabolic rate induced by thyroid hormone. When metabolic rate increases, cardiac workload increases proportionately.

a, b, and **c.** Thyroid hormone does not alter the function of the pancreas, bone marrow, or kidneys. Therefore, it would not be expected to aggravate diabetes mellitus, anemia, or renal failure.

11. **Correct answer is c.** Caffeine speeds the metabolic rate increasing body heat production.

a. Sodium intake should not be increased without consulting a physician. Excessive salt intake can produce undesirable fluid shifts.

b. Exercise should be done at the coolest times of the day (e.g., early morning). Activity should be avoided in the late afternoon, which is usually the warmest part of the day.

d. Clothing should be lightweight, light colored, and loose fitting. Dark clothing retains heat.

12. **Correct answer is b.** Alcohol dilates blood vessels, increasing heat loss.

a. Working muscles produce heat, so exercise actually decreases the risk of hypothermia.

c. Hypothyroidism would increase the risk of hypothermia by decreasing the metabolic rate. Hyperthyroidism increases the metabolic rate, producing more heat.

d. NSAIDs may be used to reduce fever to normal. They do not reduce the temperature below the normal range and do not increase the risk of hypothermia.

11

Neurologic and Sensory Disorders

NURSING HIGHLIGHTS

1. The nurse should work with the families of elderly clients with neurologic problems to sustain the client's independence as much and as long as possible. Both the nurse and the family need to realize that the client can still do many things on his/her own, even if they are done slowly and awkwardly.
2. The nurse should be prepared to deal patiently with personality changes related to the client's decline in mental and physical functioning.
3. The nurse should be aware that the frustration experienced by the elderly increases with multiple sensory losses, as does the time needed to adjust to these losses.

GLOSSARY

extrapyramidal system—a part of the nervous system, made up of nuclei and fibers, that controls and coordinates motor activities
stereognosis—the ability to perceive through the sense of touch the form and nature of objects

I. Neurologic disorders

See text pages
_____

A. Age-related changes (same as section II,H of Chapter 2)

B. General nursing assessment
  1. General observation
     a) Note any asymmetry or deformity.
     b) Observe for any signs of paralysis or weakness.
     c) Listen for any problems with speech articulation (dysarthria) or language recognition and comprehension problems (dysphasia).
  2. Interview
     a) Inquire about any tingling, numbness, blackouts, headaches, twitching, seizures, dizziness, weakness, and changes in mental status or level of functioning.
     b) To test for dysphasia, ask the client to name objects in the room or, for a client with adequate visual acuity, to read and write simple sentences.
  3. Physical examination
     a) Check sensation by having the client close his/her eyes and describe sensation as you lightly touch the forehead, cheek, hands, legs, and so on.
     b) Test for stereognosis by having the client identify common objects placed in the hand while the eyes are closed.
     c) Test coordination and cerebellar functioning by having the client alternate touching your finger and his/her own nose as you reposition your finger in different areas; perform this test with both of the client's arms.
     d) Test coordination in legs by having the client, while supine, move the heel of 1 foot against the shin of the other leg.
     e) Test oculomotor nerve functioning by having the client track your finger as you move it to different points horizontally and vertically.
     f) Test facial nerve functioning by asking the client to smile, pull the mouth to each side, and lift the lips to show teeth.

C. Common disorders
  1. Parkinson's disease
     a) Definition: progressive disease of central nervous system (CNS) that affects control and movement
     b) Pathophysiology and etiology
        (1) Pathophysiology: degeneration of extrapyramidal system, reduction of dopamine levels in the corpus striatum of the brain
        (2) Etiology: cause unknown; associated with history of arteriosclerosis, encephalitis, and/or metal poisoning

        c) Symptoms: tremors (especially "pill rolling"), shuffling gait, slowing of voluntary movements, muscle rigidity and weakness, drooling, difficulty swallowing, slow speech, monotone voice, masklike facial expression; *personality changes and confusion common in the elderly*

        d) Treatment: drug therapy (levodopa, carbidopa/levodopa, anticholinergics), exercises and physical therapy to maintain joint mobility and to relieve muscle spasms and contractures

  2. Herpes zoster (shingles)

        a) Definition: acute inflammatory varicella viral infection that is contagious until the lesions dry

        b) Pathophysiology and etiology

           (1) Pathophysiology: infection of sensory nerve ganglia leading to vesicular eruptions that follow the path of the cranial, thoracic, or cervical nerves; formation of crusts after rupture of serum- and pus-filled vesicles

           (2) Etiology: reactivation of latent infection due to age-related decline in immunity; loss of immunity due to radiation, chemotherapy, or leukemia

        c) Symptoms: pain, itching, formation of vesicles (often a late symptom)

        d) Treatment: corticosteroids, analgesics, antiviral drugs (e.g., acyclovir), topical preparation (to dry lesions)

D. Essential nursing care

  1. Nursing assessment (same as section I,B of this chapter)

  2. Nursing diagnoses

        a) Impaired physical mobility related to muscle rigidity associated with Parkinson's disease

        b) Self-care deficits (feeding, bathing, dressing) related to tremors

        c) Powerlessness related to neurologic disability and dependency

        d) Ineffective individual coping related to depression about progression of Parkinson's disease

        e) Ineffective family coping related to client's dependency due to Parkinson's disease

        f) Pain related to herpes zoster infection

  3. Nursing implementation (intervention)

        a) Work with the client who has Parkinson's disease to develop a program of daily exercise and to practice walking techniques that enhance balance.

        b) Encourage the client with Parkinson's disease to obtain assistive devices (e.g., raised toilet seat, bedside rails, walker) and to use adaptive devices (e.g., Velcro closures on clothes, slip-on shoes, special utensils).

   c) Instruct the client with Parkinson's disease to allow ample time to perform activities of daily living (ADLs) and to do as much as possible himself/herself.

   d) Help the client with Parkinson's disease recognize abilities and pastimes that can still be enjoyed and encourage the client to participate in social and recreational events.

   e) Provide emotional support to the family of the client with Parkinson's disease and educate them about the disorder.

   f) Provide emotional support as the client adjusts to the limitations and adaptations that must be made as Parkinson's disease progresses.

   g) Provide analgesics as ordered to relieve pain associated with herpes zoster.

   h) Instruct the client with herpes zoster in pain-reduction techniques (e.g., meditation, relaxation therapy).

4. Nursing evaluation

   a) The client demonstrates improvement in mobility.

   b) The client recovers a degree of independence through the use of self-help equipment.

   c) The client demonstrates a positive self-concept despite limitations imposed by the disease.

   d) The client's family indicates adjustment to the client's symptoms and understands the disease better.

   e) The client with herpes zoster reports reduction of pain to tolerable levels.

5. Gerontologic nursing considerations

   a) It is more beneficial for the client to perform an action, however slowly, than to have it done by the nurse.

   b) Elderly clients with neurologic disorders are at very high risk for falls or other injuries due to dizziness, weakness, or uncoordinated movements.

   c) Because of problems with swallowing, clients with Parkinson's disease may be at risk for aspiration or choking. These clients should not eat alone.

   d) The drug regimen for a client with Parkinson's disease is complex; the family should be instructed about side effects to expect. (See section II,B,11 of Chapter 3 for side effects of antiparkinson drugs and section III,A,11 of Chapter 3 for major interactions with other drug classes.)

   e) The elderly client may need a lower-than-normal adult dose of levodopa. Levodopa should not be taken with vitamin B_6 or MAOIs (monoamine oxidase inhibitors) as the effect of levodopa is negated.

   f) A high-protein diet may antagonize the effects of antiparkinson medications.

g) The client with a neurologic disorder may vent frustration or rage at caregivers. Health care providers and family members must respond to the frustrated and irritable client with patience and tolerance, not with hurt or anger.

h) Older adults have increased incidence of neuralgia (pain) after a herpes zoster infection.

See text pages
_____

II. Sensory disorders

A. Age-related changes (same as section I,I of Chapter 2)

B. General nursing assessment
1. General observation
   a) Observe whether the client is inattentive, irritated, suspicious, or withdrawn.
   b) Look for signs of a hearing deficit.
      (1) Requests to have statements repeated
      (2) Apparent reliance on lip reading
      (3) Cocking head to hear better
      (4) Monotone or unusually loud or soft speaking voice
   c) Observe for signs of eye problems.
      (1) Apparent difficulty seeing (e.g., peering, squinting)
      (2) Abnormalities (e.g., drooping eyelids, excessive tearing or discharge, discolored sclera, unusual eye movements)
   d) Be alert for signs of diminished olfactory function (e.g., apparent unawareness of personal odors).
   e) Look for signs of diminished sensory awareness.
      (1) Burns on fingers and hands from cooking or cigarettes
      (2) Unrecognized pressure sores
      (3) Unrecognized injuries or infections of the feet
2. Interview
   a) Ask the date and extensiveness of the most recent eye and ear examinations.
   b) If eyeglasses or hearing aid is worn, ask when obtained and how (e.g., from physician, by mail order).
   c) Formulate specific questions designed to explore vision deficits or eye disease.
      (1) Changes in vision
      (2) Pain, burning, or itching in either eye
      (3) Quality of night vision
      (4) Presence of halos, flashes of light, or spots
      (5) Family history of glaucoma

d) Formulate specific questions designed to uncover ear problems or hearing loss.
   (1) Changes in hearing
   (2) Types of sounds that are harder to hear than others
   (3) Pain, itching, ringing, or a sense of fullness in the ears
   (4) Any problem with ear wax accumulation
   (5) Presence of drainage from the ears
e) Ask if the client's sense of smell has changed.
f) Ask if the client is less aware of pain or less sensitive to pressure or to the sensation of hot or cold.
3. Physical examination
   a) Eyes
      (1) Assess for alignment and symmetry.
      (2) Check for drooping eyelids, discharge, or discoloration.
      (3) Assess for dryness or excessive tearing.
      (4) Gently palpate eyeballs with lids closed for signs of high intraocular pressure (hardness) or fluid volume deficit (sponginess).
      (5) Assess pupils for size, shape, reaction to light, and ability to accommodate for near vision (PERRLA).
      (6) Test vision with an eye chart at 20 ft from the client and with different-sized type in a newspaper or by holding up fingers.
      (7) Have the client follow your finger as it moves through the visual field; note any apparent blind spots or abnormal eye movements (e.g., nystagmus).
   b) Ears
      (1) Assess for symmetry.
      (2) Inspect external ear for tenderness and masses.
      (3) With otoscope, examine ear canal for accumulation of hardened or impacted cerumen and for inflammation, discharge, and masses; note atrophy or hardening of tympanic membrane and note odor.
      (4) Check the client's ability to hear ticking watch or a whisper at a distance of about 3 inches with either ear.
      (5) With a tuning fork, assess for lateralization of sound (Weber test) and for conduction of sound (Rinne test).

C. Common disorders
   1. Vision disorders
      a) Presbyopia
         (1) Definition: inability to focus properly that often develops with age
         (2) Pathophysiology and etiology: age-related loss of elasticity of the lens of the eye and the ciliary muscles resulting in the inability of the lens to change shape for near vision
         (3) Symptoms: farsightedness
         (4) Treatment: corrective lenses

b) Cataract
   (1) Definition: a condition producing clouding of the lens of the eye or the lens capsule
   (2) Pathophysiology and etiology: age-related development of lens opacity; may be aggravated by exposure to ultraviolet rays
   (3) Symptoms: distorted vision, blurring, intolerance to bright lights; no pain or discomfort
   (4) Treatment: surgical removal of lens, followed by insertion of an intraocular lens or use of a contact lens or corrective eyeglasses

c) Glaucoma
   (1) Definition: a condition of elevated intraocular pressure within the eye
   (2) Pathophysiology and etiology: obstruction of the outflow of aqueous humor causing an increase in pressure; etiology unknown; associated with iritis, allergy, endocrine imbalance, increase in lens size, and family history of glaucoma
      (a) Acute (closed-angle) glaucoma: obstruction of aqueous humor caused by folded iris; acutely increased intraocular pressure accompanied by edema of ciliary body and dilation of pupil; blindness can occur if condition not corrected immediately
      (b) Chronic (open-angle) glaucoma: obstruction of canal of Schlemm; gradually increased intraocular pressure, with gradual impairment of peripheral vision followed by central blindness
   (3) Symptoms
      (a) Acute (closed-angle) glaucoma: severe eye pain, pupil dilation, eye redness, blurred vision, nausea, vomiting, loss of vision
      (b) Chronic (open-angle) glaucoma: loss of peripheral vision, tired feeling in eyes, headaches, halos around lights, with symptoms more noticeable in the morning
   (4) Treatment: drug therapy (e.g., carbonic anhydrase inhibitors, hyperosmotic agents, beta-adrenergic antagonists, cholinergics), surgery

d) Macular degeneration
   (1) Definition: injury or deterioration of the macula, resulting in loss of central vision
   (2) Pathophysiology and etiology: small deposits and growth of blood vessels occurring between retina and choroid;

age-related involutional degeneration or as a result of injury, infection, exudative degeneration

    (3) Symptoms: increasingly blurred central vision, difficulty reading fine print or discerning distant objects

    (4) Treatment: laser therapy; use of magnifying glasses, high-intensity reading lamps, other aids

  e) Diabetic retinopathy

    (1) Definition: deterioration of blood vessels of the retina secondary to diabetes

    (2) Pathophysiology and etiology: retinal microaneurysm followed by microinfarction and exudate formation; may progress to retinal neovascularization and retinal detachment or vitreous hemorrhage; presumably due to high glucose levels

    (3) Symptoms: blurred vision, fluctuating vision, sudden loss of vision

    (4) Treatment: control of diabetes, laser therapy

 2. Hearing disorders

  a) Presbycusis

    (1) Definition: sensorineural deafness and loss of sound discrimination resulting from aging process

    (2) Pathophysiology and etiology: changes in nerve functioning or in cochlea (e.g., hardening of cilia)

    (3) Symptoms: gradual loss of hearing beginning with higher-pitched sounds, tinnitus

    (4) Treatment: use of hearing aid

  b) Impacted cerumen

    (1) Definition: wax buildup that causes physical interference with transmission of sound waves through the ear

    (2) Pathophysiology and etiology: accumulated cerumen forming physical barrier to sound wave passage

    (3) Symptoms: partial loss of hearing, tinnitus, earache

    (4) Treatment: removal of earwax by a health care provider

  c) Otosclerosis

    (1) Definition: conduction deafness resulting from fixation of footplate of stapes

    (2) Pathophysiology and etiology: osseous growth; may progress to complete deafness

    (3) Symptoms: gradual loss of hearing in 1 or both ears, tinnitus

    (4) Treatment: stapedectomy

D. Essential nursing care

 1. Nursing assessment (same as section II,B of this chapter)

 2. Nursing diagnoses

  a) Altered sensory perception related to loss of sensory acuity

  b) Social isolation related to sensory deficit

  c) Anxiety related to inability to communicate due to sensory loss

  d) Impaired social interaction related to dislike of wearing hearing aid

e) Activity intolerance related to poor sensory ability
f) Impaired home maintenance management related to vision deficit
g) High risk for injury related to decline in vision
h) Altered nutrition, less than body requirements, related to declining sense of smell and taste

3. Nursing implementation (intervention)
   a) Work with the client to find the best correction of the sensory problem.
   b) Use aids to assist a client with a vision deficit: Help the client obtain vision aids (e.g., eyeglasses, magnifying glass) and appropriate lighting to continue enjoyed activities, see that eyeglasses are kept clean and free from breakage, label objects with large print and in bright colors, place objects where the client can find them and see that they are kept in familiar positions, announce actions in advance to prevent fear, use vivid descriptions.
   c) Assist the client in finding housekeeping assistance.
   d) Instruct the client and the family about correcting environmental hazards (e.g., loose carpeting).
   e) Use communication aids when addressing a client with a hearing deficit: Talk slowly and distinctly in a low-pitched voice, talk into the ear with less hearing loss, face the person, use gestures, write down important explanations and instructions, suggest that the client read lips.
   f) Help the client find the style and/or setting of hearing aid that is comfortable to wear and use, and be sure the aid is turned on and the batteries are in working order.
   g) For the client with a declining sense of taste or smell, plan a diet that contains foods with contrasting flavors and spices.
   h) Give emotional support and provide education to reduce frustration and aggravation.

4. Nursing evaluation
   a) The client is mastering the aids provided to him/her to reduce sensory impairment.
   b) The client's use of vision aids is allowing him/her to continue hobbies and activities.
   c) The client indicates satisfaction with assistance in cleaning and maintaining home.
   d) The client's environment has appropriate safeguards and good lighting to minimize falls and injuries.
   e) The client is eating better and finding more enjoyment in meals.

5. Gerontologic nursing considerations
    a) Because of cost, fear, or denial, elderly clients may be tolerating unnecessary decline in vision or hearing by not seeing appropriate specialist for fitting with prescription glasses or hearing aid.
    b) Clients with hearing loss can become depressed, angry, suspicious, and even paranoid in response to their inability to hear others' conversations.
    c) Clients with hearing loss may show confusion or respond inappropriately rather than acknowledge inability to hear.
    d) The elderly most commonly suffer a selective high-frequency loss rather than a general decline in hearing. They have more difficulty understanding children and women than men, and they tend to have difficulty discerning particular speech sounds, such as the consonants s, f, t, and g.
    e) Older people with diminished olfactory awareness who live alone should be advised to check shelf life on all foods to avoid eating spoiled foods and to check gas burners after use to be sure they are turned off. They should be encouraged to bathe regularly to prevent hygiene problems.

1. To test the client for dysphasia, the nurse should:
   a. Observe whether the client initiates conversation.
   b. Ask the client to repeat phrases the nurse says.
   c. Ask the client to name objects in the room.
   d. Ask the client to close his/her eyes and identify objects placed in his/her hand.

2. Facial nerve function is tested by:
   a. Watching the client smile and lift his/her lips to show the teeth.
   b. Watching eye movements as the client tracks the examiner's moving finger.
   c. Observing whether the tongue remains in midline when protruded.
   d. Touching the forehead, cheek, and chin lightly and asking what the client feels.

3. Mr. Fitz, who has Parkinson's disease, complains of difficulty performing his prescribed range-of-motion (ROM) exercises due to rigidity of his extremities. Which advice would be most helpful to him?
   a. Perform the exercises after a warm bath.
   b. Have a family member assist with the exercises.
   c. Perform the exercises immediately after awakening in the morning.
   d. Rub the muscles with an ice pack before exercising.

4. Clients being treated with antiparkinson medications to control tremors and rigidity should be advised to limit dietary intake of:
   a. Simple sugars.
   b. Protein.
   c. Sodium.
   d. Fats.

5. The most important goal of nursing care for the client with herpes zoster is:
   a. Control of drainage from lesions.
   b. Avoiding complications of bed rest.
   c. Preventing dehydration.
   d. Reduction of pain to tolerable levels.

6. Presbyopia is characterized by which of the following assessments?
   a. Nearsightedness
   b. Farsightedness
   c. Loss of depth perception
   d. Blind spots in the visual field

7. Mrs. Miller has a cataract in her left eye, for which surgery is not an option. She complains of extreme sensitivity to glare. Which advice will be most helpful to her?
   a. Keep sheer curtains over all windows.
   b. Wear an eye patch over the left eye.
   c. Use overhead lights rather than table lamps.
   d. Turn on only 1 light at a time.

8. The nurse should teach the client with glaucoma to avoid which of the following over-the-counter (OTC) medications?
   a. Aspirin
   b. Antacids
   c. Decongestants
   d. Normal saline eye drops

9. Which of the following measures would be helpful for the client with macular degeneration?
   a. Using low wattage bulbs in lamps
   b. Standing directly in front of the client while conversing
   c. Arranging all foods and utensils on 1 side of the tray
   d. Using a magnifying glass to read

10. Which of the following should be included in the nursing care plan for a client who has lost his/her sense of smell?

   a. Serve foods cold or at room temperature.
   b. Include foods with a variety of textures in each meal.
   c. Avoid the use of strong spices.
   d. Encourage the client to season foods to suit his/her tastes.

11. When speaking to an elderly client with presbycusis, the nurse should:

   a. Exaggerate lip movements.
   b. Raise the volume of the voice.
   c. Lower the pitch of the voice.
   d. Place the nurse's mouth near the client's ear.

12. Which of the following sensory assessment findings suggests impacted cerumen in the right ear?

   a. The client hears a watch tick at a distance of 3 inches.
   b. The client has trouble distinguishing consonant sounds such as s and f.
   c. When the pinna is pulled back, the client reports pain in the ear canal.
   d. Sound lateralizes to the right ear when the Weber test is performed.

ANSWERS

1. **Correct answer is c.** Asking the client to name objects indicates not only that the client can speak but that the client comprehends the meaning of the words.

   a. There might be many reasons a client does not initiate conversation. This would not be a specific test for dysphasia.
   b. Repeating phrases could be simple imitation. The client can imitate speech without comprehending it.
   d. Closing the eyes and identifying objects in the hand is a test for stereognosis, not dysphasia.

2. **Correct answer is a.** The facial nerve controls the muscles of the lips and cheek.

   b. Watching eye movements tests the oculomotor nerve.
   c. Observing position of protruded tongue tests the hypoglossal nerve.
   d. Touching the facial areas lightly tests the trigeminal nerve.

3. **Correct answer is a.** Heat relaxes muscles, reducing the rigidity. This will improve ROM and facilitate the performance of the exercises.

   b. While the muscles are rigid, an assistant will not be able to perform ROM exercises any more effectively than the client. Active ROM exercises are more effective than passive ROM exercises.
   c. Rigidity may actually be worse after the period of immobility during sleep.
   d. Ice, used to relieve pain or strengthen muscle contraction, may actually increase rigidity.

4. **Correct answer is b.** Protein interferes with the actions of many antiparkinson medications. None of the other nutrients affects Parkinson's disease or its treatment.

   a. Simple sugars should be limited for clients with diabetes.
   c and d. Sodium and fat intake should be limited for clients with cardiovascular disorders.

5. **Correct answer is d.** Herpes zoster is often extremely painful. Analgesics, relaxation techniques, and anti-inflammatory drugs may be used to reduce the pain, although complete relief may be impossible.

   a. The lesions of herpes zoster seldom produce copious drainage. Once vesicles rupture, they quickly form crusts.
   b. Bed rest is not required for herpes zoster. The client may voluntarily limit movement to avoid pain and should be encouraged to remain mobile.

c. Dehydration is not a common complication of herpes zoster.

6. **Correct answer is b.** Presbyopia is caused by decreased ability of the ciliary muscles to produce changes in lens shape to accommodate for near vision. Farsightedness is the result.

   a. Nearsightedness usually develops earlier in life, often in childhood or adolescence.
   c. Depth perception is lost when unilateral blindness occurs, as when retinal detachment, glaucoma, or cataract occurs in 1 eye.
   d. Blind spots may be caused by retinal detachment or migraine headache. Central vision is lost with macular degeneration.

7. **Correct answer is a.** Sheer draperies diffuse sunlight, reducing glare.

   b. Patching the eye would be inappropriate, as it would impair depth perception. Prolonged patching can result in complete loss of vision.
   c. Overhead lights often produce more glare than well-shaded table lamps.
   d. Multiple lamps with lower-wattage bulbs produce less glare than a single lamp with a higher-wattage bulb.

8. **Correct answer is c.** OTC decongestants are sympathomimetic drugs, which increase intraocular pressure. This would worsen the pathology of glaucoma.

   a. Aspirin does not increase intraocular pressure and is not contraindicated in glaucoma. It is contraindicated for clients taking anticoagulants.
   b. Antacids do not increase intraocular pressure and are not contraindicated for clients with glaucoma. Antacids may, however, reduce absorption of other drugs taken orally and should not be taken simultaneously with other drugs.
   d. Normal saline drops (e.g., Tears Naturale) may be used by the elderly to treat excessive dryness due to reduced tear production. The drops contain no active drugs and are not contraindicated in glaucoma. They should not be used at the same time as drugs that are given for glaucoma, however, to avoid diluting the medication.

9. **Correct answer is d.** Clients with macular degeneration often have difficulty reading fine print. Magnifying glasses help correct this problem.

   a. A high-intensity reading lamp may be helpful as central vision becomes more blurred. Use of lower-wattage bulbs is appropriate for clients with cataracts.
   b. Since central vision is most affected, positioning oneself to 1 side of the midline of the visual field may permit the client to see the speaker better.
   c. Placing food and utensils on 1 side of the food tray is appropriate for a client with a visual field cut due to a cerebrovascular accident (CVA). Central vision is most affected in macular degeneration so the client can see both sides of the tray.

10. **Correct answer is b.** Since taste is strongly dependent on smell, the client's appetite may be affected. Variety in textures may increase the appeal of meals when taste and smell are diminished.

    a. Flavors are enhanced by heating foods. Since decreased smell will decrease taste sensation, foods should be heated to increase their flavor.
    c. Spices contribute to the flavor of foods and may improve appetite when decreased smell impairs taste sensation. Pepper and curry are trigeminal nerve stimulants, offering an alternative to odors for stimulation.
    d. Clients who cannot smell often overuse salt or sugar in an effort to achieve the flavors they recall. Such overseasoning may lead to problems with blood pressure or glucose tolerance and should be discouraged.

11. **Correct answer is c.** The client with presbycusis loses the ability to hear high-pitched sounds first. Lowering the voice pitch improves the probability that the client will understand the nurse.

a and **d.** Exaggerating lip movements and placing the mouth near the client's ear would both interfere with lip reading, which the client may be using to improve comprehension, sometimes without being aware of it. Exaggerating the lip movements distorts them, and moving the mouth close to the ear moves the lips out of the client's visual field.
b. Most people raise the pitch of the voice when they raise the volume. This actually reduces the client's ability to hear what is said.

12. **Correct answer is d.** Impacted cerumen blocks transmission of background noise by air conduction, allowing the sound produced by a tuning fork held against the forehead (Weber test) to be heard in, or lateralized to, the affected ear.

a. This is a normal finding. Cerumen impaction would impair hearing of the watch tick.
b. This is consistent with presbycusis, not cerumen impaction.
c. This is consistent with inflammation in the external ear canal (e.g., "swimmer's ear").

12

Mental Disorders

NURSING HIGHLIGHTS

1. Mental health problems are often overlooked by health care providers because they are mistaken for normal responses to such aspects of aging as chronic illnesses or the deaths of spouse and friends.
2. Mental disorders are the most frequently diagnosed problems in nursing homes.
3. The nurse must treat the client who has dementia with respect, recognizing the client's worth and need for dignity.
4. The nurse working with depressed clients should empathize without identifying, to avoid the risk of becoming depressed in response.
5. The isolated elderly person, especially one grieving for a spouse or suffering another major loss, should be encouraged to form other relationships and to participate in volunteer or social activities.

6. Depression often accompanies chronic illness, disability, and nonpathologic declines in memory. Depression can retard or reduce recovery and can cause disability equal to that of major chronic illness. Education about an illness can diminish fears that may be a source of depression or anxiety.
7. Suicide is a leading cause of death in older adults, and about 25% of all suicides are committed by adults over age 65.
8. Many elderly people perceive a stigma attached to a diagnosis of mental illness. Often they are unwilling to undergo psychotherapy but will participate in a group that cannot be obviously categorized as meant for "mental patients."

GLOSSARY

agnosia—inability to recognize objects or to grasp the meaning of words, objects, or symbols

anhedonia—inability to experience happiness from normally pleasurable experiences

aphasia—loss of language ability; inability to remember correct name for an object or a person

apraxia—inability to perform purposeful movements

confabulation—the act of making up information to cover memory loss

crystallized intelligence—mental ability that consists of using past learning and experiences for problem solving

fluid intelligence—mental ability that involves emotions, retention of nonintellectual information, creative capabilities, spatial perceptions, and aesthetic appreciation

lipofuscin—abnormal granular pigment associated with the oxidation of unsaturated lipids that, when present in excessive amounts, interferes with the transport of essential metabolites and information-bearing molecules

neuritic plaques—accumulations of the protein amyloid surrounded by abnormal dendrites and axons of nerve cells

neurofibrillary tangles—abnormal entwined filaments within a neuron; found mainly in the part of the brain responsible for short-term memory and emotion

ENHANCED OUTLINE

I. Age-related changes

A. Physiologic changes in the brain
    1. Loss of neurons (about 20%) in cerebral cortex; no loss of brainstem nerve cells
    2. Decrease in brain weight and size (about 7%) due to the decrease in cortical volume

See text pages
_____

3. Appearance of neuritic plaques and neurofibrillary tangles in advanced old age or with Alzheimer's disease
4. Accumulation of lipofuscin

B. Changes in intellectual functioning
1. No change to basic intelligence (verbal and math skills)
2. Decline in short-term, or recent, memory
3. Increased retrieval time needed for long-term memory
4. Distractibility increased during performance of complex intellectual tasks
5. Greater difficulty in extinguishing old responses and learning new ones
6. Greater difficulty with perceptual motor tasks
7. Decline in fluid intelligence while crystallized intelligence stays constant or continues to develop

C. Psychosocial changes
1. No change in basic personality traits
2. Possible alterations in self-concept due to stressful life events and role changes

II. General nursing assessment

See text pages
_____

A. General observation
1. Observe the client's overall grooming, and note whether the clothing is clean, appropriate to the season and occasion, and correctly worn.
2. Observe any unusual movement patterns or posture, including tongue rolling, twitching, tremors, and hand wringing or writhing.
3. Observe the client's affect, including a flat affect or masklike facial expression or inappropriate expressions of fear or anger.
4. Observe level of consciousness, noting evidence of lethargy or stupor.
5. Listen carefully to speaking style, noting the use of appropriate and articulate responses, garbled speech, incorrect word choices, or word-finding difficulties.
6. Observe any abnormal slowing of speech and movement that is unrelated to physical illness.
7. Notice any signs of agitation in facial expression, movements, and speech.
8. Pay attention to statements expressing worthlessness, guilt, or hopelessness.

9. Take note of any suicidal ideation such as statements about wishing to die, being better off dead, or not deserving to live.
10. Notice any obsessive or ritually repeated behavior.

B. Interview
　1. Cognitive testing
　　a) Orientation: Ask name, date, time, and season; ask the client to identify where she/he is.
　　　(1) Self-knowledge of one's identity is a significant indicator of cognitive function.
　　　(2) Tests of cognitive ability include the Mini-Mental State Examination (see Chapter 2, Figure 2-4), the Short Portable Mental Status Questionnaire, and the Set Test.
　　b) Recall: At the beginning of the interview, ask the client to repeat the names of 3 common objects and to remember them; later in the interview, ask the client to recall them.
　　c) 3-stage command: Ask the client to perform 3 simple related tasks (e.g., to pick up a piece of paper, fold it once, and hand it to you).
　　d) Reasoning: Ask the client to explain the meaning of a common phrase or proverb (e.g., a rolling stone gathers no moss).
　　e) Concentration: Ask the client to count backwards from 100 in 7's (if the client has sufficient education level). If the client cannot do the serial 7's test, simplify the task to counting by 5's or 2's.
　　f) Calculating ability: Ask the client to solve simple math problems (e.g., If 4 tomatoes cost $1.00, how many tomatoes can you buy for $3.00?).
　　g) Discontinue testing if the client is incapable of responding or becomes upset.
　2. General questions: to be asked of family members if the client is unable to respond
　　a) Take medical history.
　　　(1) Presence of physical illness
　　　(2) Dietary habits
　　　(3) History of vision and hearing impairments
　　　(4) History of head trauma
　　　(5) Alcohol consumption
　　　(6) Use of prescriptions, over-the-counter (OTC) drugs, herbal medicines, family remedies, and psychoactive substances
　　b) Obtain work and social histories to determine prior level of functioning.
　　c) Obtain a family history of mental illness.
　　d) Determine the length and approximate date of onset of the present illness and whether the onset was rapid or gradual.

e) Ask specific questions about symptoms of the present condition (e.g., changed patterns in diet, sleep, concentration, memory, and sexual function and interest).

f) Inquire whether there was a precipitating event (e.g., major illness, loss of spouse).

g) Ask whether there have been past occurrences and if the client has ever been hospitalized for a mental illness.

h) If the client expresses hopelessness, determine whether the client has thoughts of suicide and whether he/she has a plan for carrying it out.

C. Physical examination

1. Conduct a complete physical examination.

a) To identify any underlying physical disorder (e.g., systemic infection, endocrine disorders, cardiac function, neurologic deficits, hypoglycemia, hyperthermia)

b) To determine whether generalized complaints of poor health or pain have a physiologic basis or might be somatic indicators of depression

2. Note any injury or scarring that might indicate a suicide attempt.

III. Common disorders

See text pages
_____

A. Cognitive disorders

1. Delirium

a) Definition: disturbed cognition evidenced by acute confusional or stuporous state; usually rapid onset, brief course, and reversible (see Nurse Alert, "Main Differences between Delirium and Dementia")

b) Pathophysiology and etiology: cerebral impairment; usually has specific organic cause (e.g., medical disorder, alcohol intoxication, drug toxicity, systemic infection, withdrawal from drugs, reaction to certain medications, inadequate oxygenation, electrolyte imbalances, postoperative states, sensory deprivation, sensory overload)

c) Symptoms

(1) Behavioral: restlessness and apprehension (early signs that may be missed or attributed to confusion); clouded consciousness; fluctuating levels of intensity and awareness; disorientation to time, place, and person; incoherent speech and perceptual disturbances (e.g., illusions, hallucinations); mood swings (e.g., agitation/apathy); impulsive actions; disordered thought

        (2) Physical: tremors, elevated pulse and respiration, temperature changes, fatigue

    d) Treatment: identification and correction of the underlying disorder

2. Dementia

    a) Definition: a progressive, usually irreversible impairment in intellectual functioning, usually with specific deterioration in memory, judgment, and capacity for abstract thought and with personality changes; may be primary (e.g., Alzheimer's disease, multi-infarct dementia) or secondary to infection (e.g., HIV), head trauma, metabolic disturbances (e.g., thyroid dysfunction), folic acid or vitamin B_{12} deficiency, or adverse effects of a drug; approximately 80% of dementias in the elderly are primary

    b) Pathophysiology and etiology

        (1) Multi-infarct dementia: multiple occlusions of small cerebral arteries, resulting in irreversible tissue damage

        (2) Alzheimer's disease: atrophy of associational areas of the brain, disruptions of the neurotransmitters acetylcholine and serotonin, and formation of neuritic plaques and neurofibrillary tangles; course of 1–10 years with death usually due to infection, malnutrition, or dehydration; cause unknown, but may be related to genetics, virus, autoimmune defects, or accumulation of protein or aluminum in the brain

    c) Symptoms

        (1) General: memory loss; confusion; inability to plan, abstract, or sequence; labile affect

        (2) Additions with multi-infarct dementia: weak extremities, gait abnormalities, exaggerated deep-tendon reflexes

        (3) Mild or early symptoms
           (a) Ability to live independently but with difficulty at work and some social impairment (e.g., trouble identifying people and balancing checkbook, indifference to courtesy and social ritual)
           (b) Forgetting appointments, misplacing objects
           (c) Depression or anxiety due to awareness of deteriorating faculties
           (d) Use of confabulation
           (e) Need for frequent checks to be sure of functioning
        (4) Moderate-stage symptoms
           (a) Decline in memory, especially of recent events, and slowing in response
           (b) Disorientation and difficulties following simple directions and understanding everyday events
           (c) Neglect of hygiene, nutrition, and safety
           (d) Wandering
           (e) Progressive paranoia, hallucinations, agitation, nocturnal restlessness, and insomnia
           (f) Increasing agnosia, aphasia, and apraxia
        (5) Severe-stage symptoms
           (a) Progression of difficulty communicating, leading to incoherence or muteness
           (b) Inability to participate in self-care
           (c) Incontinence
           (d) Confinement to bed
           (e) Stupor, coma, and death
      d) Treatment
        (1) Maintenance of optimal functioning; in moderate stage, supervision required and perhaps institutionalization; in severe stage, intensive and total care needed for nutrition, hygiene, fluids, and elimination
        (2) Administration of tacrine (Cognex)
           (a) Arrests or lessens symptoms in selected clients with mild or moderate Alzheimer's disease; does not, however, stop the destruction of brain cells
           (b) May cause side effects: liver toxicity, nausea, vomiting (frequent blood tests recommended to check liver enzyme levels)
   B. Depression
      1. Definition: affective disorder marked by excessive or persistent sadness that has increased incidence with age

2. Pathophysiology and etiology
    a) Biologic factors: imbalance in neurotransmitters and hormones
    b) Precipitating factors: illness; increasing disability; isolation; loneliness; loss of friends and loved ones, especially of a spouse; reduction in status with retirement or with reduced income and resulting feelings of powerlessness and uselessness
    c) Drug reaction: antihypertensives, antihistamines, oral hypoglycemics, hormones, barbiturates, benzodiazepines, neuroleptics, alcohol, cimetidine, levodopa, ranitidine
3. Symptoms: apathy or loss of interest in usual activities, fatigue or lethargy, anhedonia, feelings of worthlessness or hopelessness, indecisiveness, eating and sleep disorders (e.g., anorexia, early morning awakening), weight loss or gain, somatic symptoms (e.g., diffuse pain, gastrointestinal discomfort), slowed speech and thought processes, memory impairment, suicidal ideation, irritability, social withdrawal, deterioration in hygiene and grooming
4. Treatment: antidepressant drug therapy (e.g., tricyclics, MAOIs [monoamine oxidase inhibitors]), psychotherapy, group therapy, family therapy, electroconvulsive therapy

C. Anxiety
1. Definition: a state of prolonged alarm, a feeling of stress and emotional disturbance based on a perceived threat to well-being
2. Pathophysiology and etiology: stimulation of the sympathetic nervous system that produces physiologic changes (e.g., increase in blood pressure, pulse, respirations; frequency of urination), along with perceptual, cognitive, and behavioral changes; in the elderly, often in response to the weakened condition and diminished ability to defend oneself that often accompanies aging or in response to the inability to understand one's environment (especially in a nursing home)
3. Symptoms: insomnia, fatigue, restlessness, confusion, rigidity in thinking or behavior, somatic complaints
4. Treatment: anxiolytic medication (e.g., benzodiazepines), biofeedback therapy, relaxation therapy (especially breathing exercises)

D. Paranoia
1. Definition: delusions of persecution or abnormal suspiciousness of others' intentions; paranoia of late life onset is sometimes called paraphrenia
2. Pathophysiology and etiology: diverse; related to decline in sensory acuity, especially hearing loss, which results in confusion and misinterpretations, and to feelings of insecurity due to disability, isolation, illness, or financial constraints
3. Symptoms: hostility, uncooperativeness, irritability, refusal to sleep or eat, withdrawal
4. Treatment: clear consistent explanations and responses that do not support delusions

See text pages

IV. Essential nursing care

A. Nursing assessment (same as section II of this chapter)

B. Nursing diagnoses
   1. Altered thought processes related to hallucinations
   2. High risk for injury related to decreased cognitive functioning
   3. Anxiety related to increasing forgetfulness
   4. Self-care deficit in feeding and toileting related to cognitive impairment
   5. High risk for fluid volume deficit related to forgetfulness or loss of self-care skills
   6. Impaired verbal communication related to aphasia
   7. Ineffective individual coping related to anger resulting from feelings of powerlessness and abandonment
   8. Altered nutrition, less than body requirements, related to anorexia of depression
   9. Hopelessness related to poor health and nursing home residence
   10. Self-care deficit in bathing and hygiene related to depression
   11. Dysfunctional grieving related to loss of spouse
   12. High risk for trauma related to suicidal ideas and impulses
   13. Sleep pattern disturbance related to anxiety or paranoia
   14. Impaired social interaction related to paranoia
   15. Compromised family coping related to the client's mental condition

C. Nursing implementation (intervention)
   1. Ensure the safety of the client with a cognitive disorder.
      a) Provide continuous observation during periods of agitation.
      b) Protect the client from objects that might cause harm.
         (1) Remove toxic or inedible objects that might be ingested accidentally.
         (2) Remove matches and lighters.
         (3) Cover unused electric outlets and sockets.
         (4) Take knobs off stoves so that the client cannot turn on the burners.
         (5) Cover or remove fans and motors.
         (6) Use Plexiglas or screens in windows.
      c) Place alarms on doors to prevent wandering.
      d) Try not to leave the client alone, especially at night.
      e) Have the client wear an identification bracelet that indicates name, address, telephone number, and name of illness.

2. Address the physical well-being of the client with a cognitive disorder.
   a) Administer and monitor medications as ordered.
   b) Help the client move around the room if possible; reposition frequently to avoid pressure ulcers.
   c) Alter hygiene and grooming schedule to accommodate the client's alertness phases; provide assistance as necessary.
   d) Monitor food intake and fluid intake and output.
   e) Provide toileting assistance at regular intervals.
   f) To promote sleep, promote methods of relaxation (e.g., back rubs).
3. If possible, continually orient the client with a cognitive disorder to date, place, name, and activities of daily living (ADLs). (This is not possible with moderate and advanced Alzheimer's disease.)
4. Listen carefully to the cognitively impaired client, taking cues about what is important from the client.
   a) Attempt to find the meaning in the client's statements, even if they seem bizarre or nonsensical.
   b) Restate what you think was the main thought expressed by the client, using words such as, "You are worried about...".
5. Develop memory aids for important information (e.g., labeling rooms, drawers, and often-used objects) and give written instructions as needed so the client with a cognitive impairment can continue independent functioning.
6. Have family supply familiar and comforting belongings for the client's room.
7. Limit the negative behaviors associated with cognitive disorders (e.g., repetitive actions such as folding clothes, combativeness, agitation, biting, inappropriate sexual behavior, rummaging).
   a) Avoid activities that precipitate or promote the behavior.
   b) Find alternatives to procedures that provoke the behavior.
   c) Reinforce positive behavior.
   d) Minimize stimulation (e.g., noise, excessive light).
   e) Provide exercise as tolerated.
   f) Explain activities, and keep them simple and predictable.
   g) Relocate the client to a more private area.
8. Provide for the physical well-being of the client who is depressed.
   a) Administer and monitor medications as ordered.
   b) Provide measures to minimize anorexia, poor sleep habits, and constipation.
      (1) Weigh the client every few days.
      (2) Monitor intake and output, including bowel movements.
      (3) Offer the client foods, especially those high in fiber, that he/she likes.
      (4) Sit with the client while he/she eats.
      (5) Frequently offer the client the high-protein, high-calorie snacks and fluids that he/she likes.

      (6) When appropriate, have the client take meals in the dining room with others.

      (7) Suggest rest periods after activities.

      (8) Encourage the client not to stay in bed all day.

      (9) Help allay feelings of insecurity before bedtime; provide relaxation techniques.

    c) Establish a routine to encourage better grooming and keep the client active and involved.

9. Listen empathically and provide positive feedback to build self-esteem.

10. Respect the depressed client's personal space and needs.

11. Arrange for the client who is depressed to join a group to discuss feelings with peers and to share reminiscences to increase self-esteem and a sense of identity and personal continuity.

12. Encourage the client who is depressed to join movement therapy groups to gain the antidepressant effects of exercise and to build a sense of independence and ability.

13. For the client with suicidal tendencies, take measures to keep the client from harm (see Nurse Alert, "Identifying the Elderly Client at Risk for Suicide").

14. For the client who is experiencing anxiety, avoid overstimulation, explain all procedures before or as they are carried out, and establish a predictable routine with consistent care by a minimum number of staff.

15. For the client with paranoia, communicate in a nonthreatening, calm manner.

16. Provide emotional support and education for the family of the client who has a cognitive impairment or mood disorder.

D. Nursing evaluation

1. The client's safety is maintained.

2. The client's physical well-being is maintained.

3. If applicable, the client becomes oriented to time, place, and person.

4. The client deals with occasional forgetfulness with less emotional upset.

5. The client is involved in self-care to the extent possible.

6. The client is able to communicate with the health care staff.

7. The depressed client's self-esteem increases.

8. The client demonstrates a reduction in or elimination of suicidal thoughts.

9. The client appears less anxious.

Identifying the Elderly Client at Risk for Suicide

Depression is believed to be a cause in one-half to two-thirds of the suicides among the elderly. A type of benign suicide, in which elderly adults literally give up, may account for many of the deaths that occur within the first year of residence in a nursing home. Overt suicide attempts tend to be well planned by older adults and are likely to be successful on the first try.

Triggering events

- Severe illness
- Entering a nursing home
- Death of a loved one
- Anniversary of the death of a loved one
- Loneliness
- Retirement

Warning signs

- Refusing food
- Refusing treatment
- Withdrawal from family or social relationships
- Refusing, misusing, or hoarding medications
- Taking unusual risks
- Giving away cherished belongings
- Evidence of a suicide plan and the means to carry it out
- Apparent sudden recovery from depression (may indicate that the client has become goal-directed enough to formulate and carry out a suicide plan)

Precautions

- Control access to sharp objects.
- Keep windows locked.
- For inpatients, check the mouth to be sure each dose of antidepressant medication has been swallowed and not hoarded.
- For severely depressed outpatients, give only a 1-week supply of antidepressants to prevent overdosing.
- Ask the client you believe is contemplating suicide if he/she has thought of harming himself/herself. This may lessen the person's anxiety.
- Elicit from the client a verbal or written contract not to commit suicide between each of your meetings.

10. The client experiences adequate duration of uninterrupted sleep.
11. The client with paranoia becomes less suspicious.
12. The client's family verbalizes a better understanding of and ability to cope with the client's mental condition.

E. Gerontologic nursing considerations
  1. Reversible delirium that is not treated because of being mistaken for general confusion in the elderly can lead to irreversible dementia. Failure to recognize delirium may result in failure to treat serious physiologic problems leading to death or disability.
  2. Clients with dementia can have what are known as catastrophic reactions—overwhelmed, disorganized responses to minor stresses such as overstimulation, failure, and fatigue. Provision of rest periods (e.g., quiet time, naps) reduces the incidence of catastrophic responses.
  3. Nursing home staff frequently notice a deterioration (e.g., agitation, disorientation) in their cognitively impaired clients after the sun goes down (see Nurse Alert, "Managing Sundown Syndrome").

! NURSE *ALERT* !

Managing Sundown Syndrome

- Turn on a light before dark and keep some form of lighting, such as night lights, on in the room.
- Check the client frequently and orient with explanations and touch.
- Provide physical activity in the afternoon to tire but not exhaust the client.
- Have familiar objects and possessions visible about the room.
- Provide adequate fluids to prevent dehydration.
- Help with toileting during evening and night as necessary.
- Provide quiet times and/or naps during the day to prevent exhaustion of coping reserves.
- Reduce demands on problem solving and memory functions in the evening (e.g., assist with ADLs, avoid new experiences).

How to Differentiate between Dementia and Depression

Dementia	Depression
• Usually gradual onset of symptoms	• Time of onset of symptoms usually more precisely identified than with dementia
• Attempts by the client to cover up memory loss	• No attempt by the client to hide memory loss or decreased intellectual functioning
• Anxiety about overcoming cognitive deficits	• Apathetic and no attempt to remember
• Labile affect	• Consistently depressed affect

NOTE: Depression may be present in a person who has dementia.

4. In the elderly, depression may be accompanied by a slowing and deterioration in mental functioning that can be mistaken for dementia (see Nurse Alert, "How to Differentiate between Dementia and Depression").

V. Psychotropic medication management for the elderly client

A. Antidepressants, antianxiety drugs, and sedatives and hypnotics
   1. Side effects are the primary consideration in choosing one of these drugs for the elderly client. (See Chapter 3 for drug effects and interactions.)
   2. The elderly client is at high risk for paradoxical reactions to antianxiety drugs (e.g., increased excitability, hostility, rage, confusion, hallucinations); short-acting benzodiazepines are preferred to long-acting ones, and barbiturates should be avoided. Nonpharmacologic treatments for anxiety and insomnia should be tried first. Antianxiety drug therapy should be used short-term only.

B. Antipsychotic agents
   1. The elderly client is at high risk for extrapyramidal side effects.
      a) Tardive dyskinesia is the most severe and possibly irreversible (see Nurse Alert, "Symptoms of Tardive Dyskinesia").
      b) Risk of extrapyramidal symptoms is increased with haloperidol, a high-potency antipsychotic drug that is often used for the elderly because the drug causes less orthostatic hypotension and fewer anticholinergic side effects than low-potency antipsychotic agents.

See text pages
_____

2. Elderly women are at high risk for agranulocytosis, a potentially fatal side effect of traditional neuroleptics (see Nurse Alert, "Signs of Agranulocytosis").

C. Nursing interventions
  1. Monitor for side effects that may reduce the effectiveness of a psychotropic drug and/or exacerbate behavior for which the drug was given.

! NURSE *ALERT* !

Symptoms of Tardive Dyskinesia

Watch for the following signs and symptoms of tardive dyskinesia; call them to the attention of the physician.
- Involuntary muscle spasm of fingers, toes, neck, trunk, or pelvis
- Thrusting or protruding tongue or puffed cheeks
- Lip smacking or puckering or chewing movements
- Drooling or difficulty keeping food in the mouth
- Difficulty swallowing and neck stiffness
- Facial tics and grimacing
- Eye blinking
- Slow, repetitive movements of arms and legs

NOTE: Document signs and symptoms for comparison in the future because tardive dyskinesia can develop insidiously.

! NURSE *ALERT* !

Signs of Agranulocytosis

The antipsychotic drug must be discontinued if the following signs occur:
- Infection
- High fever
- Chills
- Prostration
- Ulceration of the mucous membranes
- Sore throat
- Malaise
- White blood cell (WBC) count <500/mm^3

2. Give the lowest therapeutic dosage as ordered (30%–50% lower than for younger adults).
3. Chart behaviors related to each dose of a drug.
    a) Levels of alertness, disorientation, forgetfulness, and agitation
    b) Appropriateness of behavior
    c) Hallucinations
    d) Ability to perform ADLs
    e) Vital signs
    f) Reaction time
    g) Ability to sleep or stay awake as appropriate

1. While testing mental status, the nurse finds that the client cannot count backward from 100 by 7's. The nurse should next:

   a. Ask the client to solve a simple arithmetic problem.

   b. Ask the client to count backward from 100 by 5's or 2's.

   c. Document that the client has a deficit in concentration.

   d. Document that the client has a deficit in abstract reasoning.

2. Mr. Weller is alert and oriented to time, place, and person when admitted to the hospital with pneumonia. Four hours later the nurse finds him restless, apprehensive, and disoriented to time and place. Mr. Weller is most likely suffering from:

   a. A panic attack.

   b. Paranoia.

   c. Dementia.

   d. Delirium.

3. Which of the following is characteristic of dementia?

   a. Symptoms do not improve despite appropriate treatment.

   b. A specific physiologic cause is present.

   c. Severity of symptoms fluctuates rapidly.

   d. Significant EEG changes are seen.

4. Ms. Jackson, who has Alzheimer's disease, has been sitting in a chair near the nurses' station. She suddenly begins shouting and hitting the resident sitting next to her. Which of the following would be the best response by the nurse?

   a. Take Ms. Jackson to her room to rest.

   b. Take Ms. Jackson to the activity room to watch TV.

   c. Move the other resident to a different seat.

   d. Administer Ms. Jackson's PRN antipsychotic medication.

5. Which of the following would be appropriate to include in the nursing care plan for a client with sundown syndrome?

   a. Dim the room lights in the evening.

   b. Schedule rest periods and naps during the day.

   c. Provide mentally challenging activities to keep the client busy in the evening.

   d. Limit fluid intake in the evening.

6. The client who is receiving haloperidol (Haldol) to treat behavioral problems associated with dementia must be monitored for symptoms of tardive dyskinesia, including:

   a. Shuffling gait.

   b. Tongue chewing.

   c. Nervousness.

   d. Constant pacing.

7. To assist in monitoring for agranulocytosis in a client who receives antipsychotic medications, the nurse should check which of the following laboratory test results?

   a. White blood cell (WBC) count

   b. Hemoglobin and hematocrit

   c. Blood urea nitrogen (BUN) and creatinine

   d. Creatine phosphokinase (CPK)

8. Depressed elderly clients commonly exhibit:

   a. Agnosia.

   b. Apraxia.

   c. Aphasia.

   d. Anhedonia.

9. Which of the following should be included in the nursing care plan for an elderly client who is depressed?

   a. Minimize stimulation from bright lights or noisy environments.

   b. Assist the client to go to the dining room for meals.

   c. Perform passive range-of-motion (ROM) exercises while the client is in bed.

   d. Encourage the client to avoid contact with other depressed persons.

10. Which of the following should be recognized by the nurse as a sign that an elderly client may be planning suicide?

    a. Avoidance of risks
    b. Making a will
    c. Sudden relief of depression
    d. Increased compliance with therapy

11. Which of the following would be an appropriate outcome criterion for a client who is anxious?

    a. The client is oriented to person, place, and time.
    b. The client demonstrates improved self-esteem.
    c. The client experiences a sufficient duration of uninterrupted sleep.
    d. The client is less suspicious of staff and family.

12. Which of the following is the most appropriate nursing diagnosis for an elderly client with paranoia?

    a. High risk for trauma related to suicidal thoughts
    b. Constipation related to decreased physical activity
    c. Impaired social interaction related to misunderstanding others' intentions
    d. Hopelessness related to feelings of powerlessness

ANSWERS

1. **Correct answer is b.** The serial 7's test may be too difficult for a client whose educational level is low. The nurse should simplify the task and allow the client to try again before concluding that concentration is impaired.

   a. Solving a simple arithmetic problem tests calculation ability. When testing for concentration is complete, the nurse progresses to a different task. The client should be retested for concentration using a simpler task before proceeding to other tests.

   c. The serial 7's test does test concentration. However, the nurse should not conclude that concentration is impaired without retesting using a simpler task.
   d. Abstract reasoning is tested by asking the client to interpret a proverb.

2. **Correct answer is d.** Delirium initially produces restlessness and apprehension, which may progress rapidly to disorientation. Delirium generally has a specific organic cause, such as the fever and hypoxia that might be associated with pneumonia.

   a. Panic attacks involve sudden onset of extreme terror with physical signs of sympathetic nervous system activity (e.g., increased blood pressure, pulse; dyspnea; tremors), and they subside quickly (in 3–10 minutes). Disorientation would not be a common feature.
   b. The client with paranoia might be hostile, irritable, and uncooperative and may experience delusions of persecution. A sudden change in mental status is more likely to be related to delirium.
   c. Dementia has a gradual onset that is often not noticed initially. The earliest sign is most often memory loss.

3. **Correct answer is a.** Dementia is characterized by gradual onset, progressive deterioration, and nonfluctuating symptoms. Symptoms are usually irreversible. EEG changes are minimal.

   b, c, and **d.** These are characteristics of delirium. Delirium usually has an identifiable physiologic cause and symptoms are reversed when this cause is treated. Severity of symptoms fluctuates and EEG changes are evident in delirium.

4. **Correct answer is a.** Ms. Jackson is most likely experiencing a catastrophic reaction. She needs to be removed to a quiet place to rest.

   b. There may be other residents, unfamiliar furnishings, and multiple activities in the activity room. The extra stimulation of the TV and the surroundings will increase Ms. Jackson's confusion and agitation.

c. Moving the other resident may protect that resident, but having Ms. Jackson remain in the busy environment around the nurses' station will prolong her confusion and agitation.

d. Chemical restraint would not be the first choice. A chance to rest in a quiet environment is usually adequate to alleviate a catastrophic response.

5. **Correct answer is b.** Cognitive activities are demanding and exhausting for the client with dementia, so increased rest is needed between activities that require thinking. It is important to provide rest periods and/or naps during the day to avoid exhausting the client's coping abilities.

a. Dim light may be a trigger for sundowning behavior. Lights should be turned on in the evening, and a night light should be used throughout the night.

c. Cognitive demands must be reduced in the evening when the client is tired, to avoid catastrophic reactions to the stress of demands that exceed the client's abilities.

d. Adequate fluid intake to prevent dehydration is an important preventive measure. There is no reason to limit fluids in the evening.

6. **Correct answer is b.** Tardive dyskinesia is most often characterized by repetitive movements, especially of the face and extremities. Tongue thrusting or chewing, lip smacking, cheek puffing, and eye blinking are common.

a. A shuffling gait occurs with Parkinson's syndrome, which may also occur with antipsychotic drugs such as Haldol.

c and d. An intense internal feeling of nervousness or inability to sit still, which may be associated with pacing, reflects akathisia, another type of extrapyramidal syndrome associated with antipsychotic drug use.

7. **Correct answer is a.** Agranulocytosis is a severe decrease in the WBC count, which leaves the client vulnerable to infection. Severe sore throat, fever, and chills are additional signs.

b. Hemoglobin and hematocrit are used to monitor for anemia.

c. BUN and creatinine are used to monitor for nephrotoxicity.

d. CPK is used to detect damage to the heart or other muscles.

8. **Correct answer is d.** Anhedonia, the inability to experience happiness from normally pleasurable experiences, is an important symptom of depression.

a. Agnosia is the inability to recognize objects or to identify the meaning of words or symbols. It appears in the later stages of dementia and is not associated with depression.

b. Apraxia, the inability to perform purposeful movements, is associated with dementia, not depression.

c. Aphasia, the loss of language abilities, occurs in dementia and after some CVAs (strokes). It is not associated with depression.

9. **Correct answer is b.** The client who is depressed lacks motivation to get out of his/her room and join activities that provide contact with others. Acceptance by the group contributes to improved self-esteem. The stimulation of others' conversation and activity may improve the depressed client's mood and appetite.

a. Minimizing stimulation would be appropriate for a client with dementia. The depressed client, who may be withdrawn and apathetic, needs stimulation.

c. The depressed client needs active exercises, especially aerobic activities, which stimulate the sympathetic nervous system, increasing levels of neurotransmitters that have antidepressant effects. Passive ROM exercises do not provide this benefit, nor do they motivate the client to interact with others and get out of his/her room.

d. Depressed clients should be assisted to find peer groups in which they can discuss feelings with others. They may be more comfortable sharing feelings with people who have experienced the same kinds of difficulties.

10. **Correct answer is c.** The appearance of a sudden recovery from depression may indicate that the client has made a decision to commit suicide. True recovery from depression is usually a gradual process.

a. Unusual risk taking is a warning sign for suicide. Avoidance of risks is normal behavior in the elderly.

b. Making a will is not evidence of suicidal ideation in the elderly. It is appropriate for the elderly to make wills. Giving away cherished belongings may be a warning sign for suicide.

d. The elderly person who is considering suicide is more likely to refuse medications, treatments, or food than to become more compliant.

11. **Correct answer is c.** Sleep disturbances, such as early morning awakening, are common with anxiety. Uninterrupted sleep for a sufficient length of time would therefore indicate improvement.

a. Disorientation occurs in dementia, not anxiety. Since disorientation is not a problem for the client who is anxious, being oriented would not reflect improvement.

b. Low self-esteem occurs with depression. It is not a common sign of anxiety.

d. Suspicion of staff and family is associated with paranoia, not anxiety.

12. **Correct answer is c.** The client with paranoia may interpret attempts to provide care as threats or intent to harm him/her. The client may avoid interacting with others in order to avoid these perceived threats.

a. Suicidal ideation is common in depressed individuals, not those who are paranoid.

b. Constipation is common in depressed clients, who may stay in bed or in a chair unless encouraged by staff to be active. Constipation also occurs in late stages of dementia, when the client is unable to exercise due to muscle weakness or rigidity or apraxia.

d. Hopelessness is common in depression and in early stages of dementia, when the client is aware of progressive losses and realizes they are irreversible.

Gerontologic Nursing Comprehensive Review Questions

1. The nurse should explain to the elderly client that exercise has which of the following benefits?

   a. Delay of arthritic joint changes
   b. Reduced risk of fractures
   c. Increased respiratory residual volume
   d. Prevention of orthostatic hypotension

2. Which of the following reflects appropriate teaching to help an older adult reduce the risk of injury?

   a. Soak in a warm bath instead of using a heating pad to relieve muscular pain.
   b. Wear thong sandals ("flip-flops") instead of walking barefoot.
   c. Use high-wattage light bulbs in hallways and stairwells.
   d. Wear long robes or nightgowns to protect the legs and feet from drafts.

3. Which of the following age-related changes should the nurse expect to find in a healthy elderly person?

   a. Higher resting pulse rate
   b. Decreased cardiac output
   c. An enlarged heart
   d. Ischemic changes in the electrocardiogram (ECG)

4. When performing the psychosocial assessment of a healthy elderly client, the nurse is likely to find that:

   a. The client is easily distracted by noise and activity.
   b. The client attempts to conceal certain personality traits.
   c. The client's affect may shift rapidly without changes in stimuli.
   d. The client devotes less effort to dress and grooming than younger clients.

5. An elderly client's compliance with the drug regimen is most likely to be improved if the nurse:

   a. Describes the schedule for administration in relation to mealtimes.
   b. Reduces the amount of printed information given about each medication.
   c. Provides specific individual instructions about how to take each medication.
   d. Provides a verbal explanation of the medication regimen in addition to written instructions.

6. Signs of alcohol abuse in the elderly client include:

   a. Poor kidney function.
   b. Peripheral neuropathy.
   c. Compulsive behaviors.
   d. Constipation.

7. A hospitalized elderly client is at greatest risk to become confused or disoriented when the client:

   a. Has multiple sensory impairments.
   b. Is experiencing exacerbation of a chronic illness.
   c. Has had no previous health problems.
   d. Requires elective surgery.

8. The nurse should encourage family members who are planning to place a client in long-term care to investigate whether:

   a. The facility has a physician present at all times.
   b. Staff are able to provide total care for all residents.
   c. The facility prevents pressure sores and falls for all residents.
   d. The facility is clean and free of unpleasant odors.

9. During the initial assessment of 85-year-old Ms. Giovi, it is noted that she tends to cling to the nurse. It would be important for the nurse to assess for additional signs of:
   a. Physical neglect.
   b. Psychologic neglect.
   c. Physical abuse.
   d. Psychologic abuse.

10. Which of the following would fall within legal and ethical guidelines for care of a 95-year-old client who appears to be near death?
   a. Administration of sufficient analgesic to control pain despite associated respiratory depression
   b. Discontinuing intravenous (IV) fluids when they are unlikely to be curative
   c. Reducing frequency of monitoring to avoid having to perform CPR when a no-code order has not been written
   d. Encouraging the family to withhold consent for measures that will prolong life

11. Mr. Jackson is being treated for hypertension with thiazide diuretics. The nurse should instruct him to add potassium to his diet by increasing his intake of:
   a. Skim milk.
   b. Whole wheat bread.
   c. Spinach.
   d. Canned tuna.

12. When assessing the client's risk for a peripheral vascular disorder, the nurse should ask:
   a. Whether the client's occupation required frequent or prolonged walking.
   b. Whether the client wears garters or stockings with elastic bands.
   c. How much sodium the client consumes on an average day.
   d. Whether the client has experienced itching of the extremities.

13. In interpreting the arterial blood gas results of an 86-year-old client without known respiratory disease, which of the following would be considered a significant abnormality?
   a. Oxygen saturation 93%
   b. Blood oxygen (PO_2) 75 mm Hg
   c. Blood carbon dioxide (PCO_2) 52 mm Hg
   d. pH 7.42

14. The elderly client for whom isoniazid (INH) is prescribed to treat tuberculosis (TB) should be taught to:
   a. Consume more liver and whole wheat products.
   b. Consume more orange juice and bananas.
   c. Avoid dark green leafy vegetables.
   d. Avoid dairy products and antacids.

15. The elderly client with dysphagia should be advised to:
   a. Thin all solid foods with appropriate liquids.
   b. Tip the chin toward the chest while swallowing.
   c. Exhale completely and hold the breath while swallowing.
   d. Avoid taking fluids at mealtimes.

16. Ms. Phillips complains that she "can't get to the bathroom in time," causing her to be incontinent of urine. The nurse should identify which type of incontinence?
   a. Stress
   b. Overflow
   c. Urge
   d. Functional

17. To help slow the rate of bone loss in the elderly client, the nurse should suggest which of the following snacks?
   a. A spinach salad
   b. A cup of yogurt
   c. A roast beef sandwich
   d. Carrot and celery sticks

18. When the goal is to maintain a moist wound environment, the most appropriate treatment for a pressure ulcer would be:
    a. Wet-to-dry dressings.
    b. Enzymatic ointments.
    c. Gelfoam packing.
    d. Transparent film dressings.

19. Which of the following assessments suggests the possibility of diabetes mellitus in the elderly client?
    a. Decreased urine output
    b. Shuffling gait
    c. Obese trunk and thin extremities
    d. Genital itching

20. During very cold weather, elderly clients should be advised to:
    a. Wear a sweater under the other clothing.
    b. Have a glass of wine at bedtime.
    c. Use an electric heater in the bedroom while sleeping.
    d. Wear caps or head scarves indoors.

21. Which of the following gait assessments would be typical of the client with Parkinson's disease?
    a. Knee raised high and foot slapped down
    b. Feet placed far apart with staggering
    c. Dragging of the feet, which causes stumbling
    d. Small, shuffling steps that start slow, then increase

22. Which of the following is most likely to be seen in the elderly client with hearing loss?
    a. Refusal to speak
    b. Speaking more softly than usual
    c. Suspiciousness of family and staff
    d. Increased talkativeness

23. The nurse should advise family members who are caring for a client with dementia at home to:
    a. Confine the client to his/her bedroom at night.
    b. Administer a mild sedative in the evening.
    c. Restrain the client in a comfortable chair during periods of confusion.
    d. Remove the knobs from the stove.

24. Which of the following is consistent with a diagnosis of depression in an elderly client?
    a. The client tries to conceal memory loss.
    b. When asked to perform cognitive tasks, the client becomes anxious.
    c. Severity of the symptoms varies at different times.
    d. The client can identify rather precisely when the symptoms began.

ANSWERS

1. **Correct answer is b.** By promoting the movement of calcium into bones, exercise minimizes loss of bone mass, reducing the risk of fractures.

   a. Exercise does not delay arthritic changes. Too strenuous exercise can actually accelerate these changes.
   c. Exercise increases vital capacity. By promoting adequate exhalation, exercise actually decreases residual volume.
   d. Postural changes in blood pressure are not eliminated by exercise.

2. **Correct answer is c.** Visual impairments make dim lighting a serious hazard for the elderly. High-wattage bulbs will improve the client's ability to see hazards in these areas.

   a. Soaking in warm baths may cause circulatory changes that put excessive demands on the cardiovascular system, resulting in hypotensive episodes, with dizziness or fainting.

b. The elderly should not walk barefoot since decreased sensory function may cause injury to go unnoticed. However, loose footwear like thong sandals or slippers may cause the older person to trip and fall.

d. Long robes, gowns, or trousers also trip the older person, especially while climbing stairs.

3. **Correct answer is b.** Normal age-related changes, such as loss of contractile strength of heart muscle and decreased stroke volume, result in decreased cardiac output.

a. Changes in the sinoatrial (SA) node, the heart's natural pacemaker, commonly result in a slight reduction in resting heart rate in the elderly.

c. The healthy heart does not become enlarged and may even become smaller with loss of muscle fibers. On an x-ray the heart may appear larger as other thoracic structures narrow.

d. Ischemic changes are abnormal and indicate cardiovascular disease.

4. **Correct answer is a.** A typical age-related reaction in elderly clients is that they are more easily distracted by environmental factors, such as noise or the presence of many people, than younger clients.

b. The elderly often become increasingly open and honest in expression of their personality traits.

c. Elderly clients are as appropriate in their affect as younger ones, unless their control is impaired by disease processes, such as stroke.

d. Elderly clients do not normally lose interest in dress and grooming. Such a change would reflect pathology.

5. **Correct answer is d.** All written instructions should be discussed verbally to clarify any misunderstandings.

a. Planning medication administration around usual mealtimes may not work for elderly clients, who may not eat 3 meals or who may not eat at common mealtimes.

b. To assist memory, clients should be given sufficient written information to cover all aspects of the medication regimen.

c. The client who takes multiple medications may become frustrated by attempting to coordinate multiple individual instructions. When possible, each administration instruction should cover multiple medications.

6. **Correct answer is b.** Alcohol is neurotoxic. Long-term effects of excessive alcohol use include peripheral neuropathy, memory loss, and cerebrovascular disease.

a. Alcohol use is not commonly associated with renal damage. Liver and cardiac problems are more likely.

c. Depression is commonly associated with alcohol abuse in the elderly. Compulsive behavior is more likely to occur with other mental health problems.

d. Alcohol is more likely to produce gastritis, ulcers, or gastrointestinal (GI) bleeding than altered bowel elimination patterns.

7. **Correct answer is a.** Sensory impairments may distort the client's perceptions of the environment, making it difficult to adjust to hospital routines.

b. The client who is being treated for a chronic illness is likely to have experienced similar problems and treatments before. Familiarity with some of the care reduces the risk of confusion.

c. Although first-time hospitalizations may produce confusion, the absence of cognitive or sensory impairments in the healthy individual reduces the risk.

d. Because elective surgery permits time for preoperative preparation, the risk of confusion due to surgery-related medications, pain, and restricted mobility is limited.

8. **Correct answer is d.** A facility that has adequate staff and is well maintained will appear clean and be free of the odors of bodily wastes or spoiled food.

   a. Having a physician present at all times would be an unrealistic expectation. Long-term care does not require continuous availability of physicians on the premises. The client's physician should be reachable by telephone if needed.
   b. It is inappropriate to provide total care for all clients. Each resident should be encouraged to be as independent as possible in activities of daily living (ADLs) and decision making. The facility should provide support services to promote such independence (e.g., physical therapy, occupational therapy).
   c. It is impossible to prevent all undesirable outcomes. Incidence of pressure sores and falls should be low, but clients and families need to recognize that when a client's rights are respected appropriately and independence is promoted, some clients will fall sometimes. A better criterion would be that injuries are minimal when clients do fall; this would indicate that adequate precautions to prevent injury are being taken.

9. **Correct answer is b.** Clinging to health care professionals is a sign of psychologic neglect.

   a. Physical neglect would be suggested by delays in seeking treatment, poor hygiene, or nutritional deficits.
   c. Physical abuse is suggested by emotional lability, nervousness, passivity, or injuries consistent with traumatic handling.
   d. Psychologic abuse is suggested by clinging to the abuser, ambivalence toward caregivers, or threatening behaviors by the abuser.

10. **Correct answer is a.** Comfort measures should be provided to the client as needed. In the terminal situation, side effects such as respiratory depression must be evaluated in relation to overall quality of life.

    b. Discontinuing life-sustaining treatments such as IV fluids raises serious ethical and legal concerns.
    c. Reducing vigilance or responding slowly to a life-threatening situation (e.g., the so-called slow code) may be legally considered negligence or abandonment of the client.
    d. The health care team may not ethically play an active role in decisions about life-sustaining treatments. The health care provider should provide information about all options but not advocate for any specific option.

11. **Correct answer is a.** One and one-half cups of milk provides 600 mg of potassium (⅓ of the amount needed to replace diuretic-induced losses).

    b. Whole grain products provide B vitamins and fiber but are not high in potassium.
    c. Spinach is a good source of vitamin K, not potassium. This is a common error because the chemical symbol for potassium is K^+.
    d. Meats and fish are not good sources of potassium. Good potassium sources are generally fruits and vegetables.

12. **Correct answer is b.** Garters and elastic bands on stockings constrict blood vessels, partially obstructing blood flow. This increases the risk of peripheral vascular disease.

    a. Standing or sitting in the same position for long periods increases the risk of peripheral vascular disease. Walking decreases the risk.
    c. High sodium intake is significant in hypertension or congestive heart failure (CHF). High fats and cholesterol are risk factors for peripheral vascular disease.
    d. Itching might occur with dry skin, which may develop secondary to a peripheral vascular disorder. Itching is not a common sign of peripheral vascular disease, however.

13. **Correct answer is c.** The partial pressure of CO_2 should remain within the same parameters as for younger clients (35–46 mm Hg).

   a. Oxygen saturation in the elderly is often reduced to 93%–94%; 93% would not be a significant abnormality.
   b. Partial pressure of O_2 in the elderly often drops to 75–80 mm Hg; 75 mm Hg would not be a significant abnormality.
   d. The normal parameters for pH (7.35–7.45) do not change for the elderly; a result of pH 7.42 is within the normal range.

14. **Correct answer is a.** Meats, especially liver, and whole grains, especially wheat germ and wheat bran, are good sources of pyridoxine (vitamin B_6). Pyridoxine should be increased to help prevent peripheral neuropathy due to INH effects.

   b. Orange juice and bananas are good sources of potassium and would be indicated for clients receiving thiazide or loop diuretics.
   c. Avoiding dark green leafy vegetables would be appropriate for clients receiving oral anticoagulants who should decrease vitamin K intake.
   d. Clients taking tetracyclines should avoid dairy products and antacids.

15. **Correct answer is b.** Tipping the chin toward the chest while swallowing assures that the epiglottis closes completely, preventing aspiration.

   a. Thinning solid foods is appropriate for acute painful conditions such as tonsillitis. In the elderly, dysphagia is most often related to muscle weakness or rigidity, and liquids are the most difficult items to swallow. Most elderly clients with dysphagia benefit from thickening liquids.
   c. The client should inhale before each swallow. The danger of aspiration increases if the client inhales too quickly after a swallow. Exhaling before swallowing increases the risk of inhaling while food is in the esophagus.

   d. Avoiding fluids at meals would be appropriate for a client with dumping syndrome. It is not helpful for dysphagia.

16. **Correct answer is c.** Urge incontinence, caused by irritation or spasm of the bladder wall, causes sudden elimination of urine immediately after awareness of the need to void. The client often reports that he/she "can't reach the bathroom in time."

   a. Stress incontinence, caused by weak pelvic muscles, results in involuntary passage of small amounts of urine whenever intra-abdominal pressure increases (e.g., laughing, coughing, sneezing, lifting).
   b. Overflow incontinence, which is associated with obstructive problems or overfilling of the bladder due to the failure of bladder muscles to contract, produces dribbling of small amounts of urine at intervals. The client may complain of frequency or a sense of abdominal or pelvic fullness. Overflow incontinence is distinguished from stress incontinence by the fact that episodes are not directly associated with an increase in intra-abdominal pressure.
   d. Functional incontinence occurs when cognitive or physical deficits prevent self-toileting. It is recognized by the passage of the usual amount of urine for a single voiding at the client's usual frequency and is validated by identifying the functional problem (e.g., inability to manage fasteners on clothing or to find the bathroom).

17. **Correct answer is b.** A cup of yogurt contains 415 mg of calcium, providing a significant portion of the recommended daily intake (800 mg for males, 1000 mg for females on estrogen, and 1500 mg for females not on estrogen).

   a. Spinach would provide iron and fiber, which do not contribute to maintenance of bone structure.
   c. Although roast beef provides protein, which helps maintain musculoskeletal

structure, it is not high in calcium, an even more essential nutrient.

d. Raw carrots and celery are high in fiber and vitamin A, which do not contribute to bone structure.

18. **Correct answer is d.** Transparent films and hydrocolloid wafers protect the wound while maintaining a moist wound surface to promote healing.

    a. Wet-to-dry dressings are used for mechanical debridement of the ulcer.

    b. Enzymatic creams and ointments are used for chemical debridement of the ulcer.

    c. Gelfoam packing is used to absorb drainage from ulcers that produce large amounts of exudate or to facilitate the growth of new cells (granulation) within the wound.

19. **Correct answer is d.** Itching of the female genitalia may be associated with chronic monilial infection, which is often associated with elevated blood glucose. The elderly may not report this sign, believing it to be a normal part of the aging process.

    a. Increased urine output (polyuria) is a sign of increased blood glucose. When blood glucose exceeds renal threshold levels, glucose is excreted in urine, producing osmotic diuresis.

    b. Shuffling gait is associated with parkinsonism. Gait changes in diabetes mellitus would be related to peripheral neuropathy, which causes stumbling or dragging of the feet.

    c. Obese trunk and thin extremities are signs of Cushing's syndrome, which is associated with prolonged steroid use. Obesity associated with diabetes mellitus is generalized, not limited to the trunk.

20. **Correct answer is d.** From 10%–30% of the normal heat loss from the body is via the head. Covering the head contributes significantly to retaining body heat.

    a. Layering clothing is a good idea, but the lightest layers should be next to the skin, with heavier clothing, like sweaters, on top.

    b. Alcohol dilates blood vessels, increasing heat loss. It should be avoided, especially at bedtime. Vasodilation provides a sensation of warmth, making the person feel warmer temporarily.

    c. Space heaters and electric heaters should never be left unattended. They should not be used near papers or bedding and should be turned off while asleep, to reduce fire risk.

21. **Correct answer is d.** Small, mincing steps that start slow and then increase in speed are typical of the gait of a client with Parkinson's disease. As bradykinesia progresses, the gait becomes slow and rigid, with lateral shifts when trying to initiate movement.

    a. Walking with the knee raised high and foot slapped down is typical of the client with footdrop.

    b. Feet placed far apart with staggering is typical of cerebellar disorders.

    c. Foot dragging is typical of peripheral neuropathy.

22. **Correct answer is c.** As hearing loss develops, the client has increasing difficulty understanding the speech of others. The client may conclude that people are deliberately speaking softly so he/she will not hear what they say and may become suspicious of their conversations.

    a and **d.** The client may increase or decrease talkativeness as hearing is lost, but changes in the quantity of speech are not as common as suspiciousness.

    b. More commonly the client with hearing loss speaks louder, since he/she does not perceive the volume of his/her voice accurately.

23. **Correct answer is d.** Removing the knobs from the stove will prevent the client from turning burners on and starting fires. Matches and lighters should also be removed and electric outlets should be covered.

a. It is best not to leave the client alone, especially at night. Confining the client in a room may increase his/her anxiety. In efforts to escape the client might be injured.

b. Clients with dementia often have paradoxical responses to medications and might become more agitated if given sedatives. Sedatives also cause confusion, which would increase safety risks.

c. Restraining the client would lead to increased anxiety and confusion and might contribute to distrust of the caregivers.

24. **Correct answer is d.** The time of onset of symptoms is usually more precisely identified in depression than in dementia.

a and **b.** The client with dementia tries to hide memory loss and is anxious about overcoming cognitive deficits. The client who is depressed is apathetic and does not try to remember information or to hide memory or cognitive problems.

c. The level of symptoms varies in the client who is delirious. Clients with dementia exhibit labile affect. The client with depression shows a consistently depressed affect.